Fattitudes

Beat Self-Defeat and Win Your War with Weight

JEFFREY R. WILBERT, PH.D.
AND
NOREAN K. WILBERT, B.S.N., R.N., C.H.E.

St. Martin's Paperbacks

FATTITUDES

Copyright © 2000 by Jeffrey R. Wilbert and Norean K. Wilbert.

"Fattitudes" is a registered trademark of Jeffrey R. Wilbert, Ph.D.

All rights reserved. No part of this book may be used or reproduced in any manner whatsoever without written permission except in the case of brief quotations embodied in critical articles or reviews. For information address St. Martin's Press, 175 Fifth Avenue, New York, NY 10010.

Library of Congress Catalog Card Number: 00-024803

ISBN: 0-312-97881-2

Printed in the United States of America

St. Martin's Press hardcover edition / May 2000
St. Martin's Paperbacks edition / May 2001

St. Martin's Paperbacks are published by St. Martin's Press, 175 Fifth Avenue, New York, NY 10010.

10 9 8 7 6 5 4 3 2

Praise for FATTITUDES

"A truly unique slant on 'dieting.' Medically speaking, the authors give very sound advice. The authors encourage readers to look inside themselves to find out why their overeating takes place, then suggest useful steps to overcome personal obstacles. This book is for the chronic dieter who is now ready to make a commitment to healthy living."
—Ramona Slupik, M.D., F.A.C.O.G., Assistant Professor of Gynecology and Obstetrics, Northwestern University Medical School, Medical Editor of *The American Medical Women's Association Complete Guide to Women's Health*

"*Fattitudes* is a breakthrough. If you've been on a diet more than once, before you start the next one, you need to read this book . . ."
—Paul Barclay, President, Just Results Lifestyle Studios, Inc.

"The Wilberts provide a user-friendly approach to understanding and changing the attitudes that add pounds and make losing weight so frustrating. *Fattitudes* offers readers practical help in controlling emotional eating and straightening out relationships with friends and family members who would undermine their dieting. This book will help the reader remove the psychological barriers that interfere with permanent weight loss."
—Edward Abramson, Ph.D., author of *Emotional Eating: What You Need to Know Before Starting Another Diet*

"With this book, the Wilberts are exposing one of the biggest secrets to successful weight management that has long eluded yo-yo dieters. Fortunately, they are willing to share the combination that can open the door to a healthier body weight for others. Their book gently takes its readers by the hand and leads them to disarm the dieting demons that have sabotaged their past attempts at weight loss. Having counseled people in weight management for the past twenty-five years as a Registered Dietitian, this book will now be assigned reading in my practice."
—Robyn Flipse, R.D., author of *The Wedding Dress Diet*

TO OUR CHILDREN,
ALLISON AND EVAN, WITH LOVE

CONTENTS

■

AUTHORS' NOTE

■

This book is intended for psychoeducational purposes only. Before beginning any new exercise or weight management program, you should always consult with a physician to obtain expert guidance. In addition, anyone needing to address significant emotional issues should do so with the collaboration of a qualified mental health professional, especially if you have a history of psychological difficulties. The authors and publisher disclaim liability for any adverse effects that might arise from any use or application of the material contained herein.

The clinical illustrations used in the following pages are derived from actual clients who have sought counseling through Fattitudes. Names and identifying information have been changed to protect confidentiality. In some instances, composites of clients with similar characteristics have been used.

ACKNOWLEDGMENTS

■

We'd like to express our appreciation to a number of folks who helped us along in our journey to authorhood. Our thanks go to Nora Vondrell, Brenda Yost, and Dr. Marsha Weston for their insightful comments on early drafts of the manuscript. Thanks to Jenny Palmer for her clinical assistance in building the Fattitudes program and for her infectious enthusiasm that helped propel us through the low spots. To Randy Palmer for his humor and artistry; to Kevin Lamb of the *Dayton Daily News* for his excellent article that helped bring attention to our work; and to Fran Henry of *The Cleveland Plain Dealer* for considering us newsworthy.

Our cheerleading squad, whose steadfast support has been inspiring and just plain fun, included Steve and Kim Hensley, Pat and Nancy Lytle, John and Sandy Heinz, and all the others in the gang. Our deepest affection goes to our moms, Joyce Wilbert and Norma Jean Hull, for teaching us what it's all about. We regret that our fathers and Norean's step-father passed away too soon to see this book come into being.

Jeff would like to give special thanks to his clients who agreed to let their stories be told, and especially to his Wednesday afternoon Fattitudes Group, whose openness and creativity helped in forming many of the ideas contained in the book.

Norean would like to applaud Paul Barclay, David Kessinger and Gary Rogers for their unflagging dedication to promoting health and fitness.

Finally, our greatest appreciation goes to our agent, Linda Konner, for her enthusiasm and steadfast commitment to this project. Linda found us a home with our fine editor, Heather Jackson, who with her able assistant, Ellen Smith, expertly guided us through the complex business of publishing with a combination of warmth and excitement.

We thank you all.

Fattitudes

PART I

■

A FAT BODY BEGINS
WITH A FAT HEAD

INTRODUCTION

■

WE HAVE MET
THE ENEMY

*It's ironic, but true, that the reason I doubled my body
size was so that I could disappear.*
—MARGIE, 34

Hello. My name is Jeff and I'm a clinical psychologist. My wife Norean and I want to tell you a story.

It's a story about our war with weight. It's a story about feelings and issues and how they made us both feel miserable for a long, long time. It's about knowing what to do and not being able to do it. About getting so frustrated and frantic that everything seemed futile. It's a story about fussing and fighting and trying a lot of stupid things that just made it all worse.

It's our story about how we struggled together for over twenty years trying to find an answer.

And finally did.

NOREAN: We want to tell you this story so you can learn from our mistakes. We want to teach you about how people get in their own way trying to lose weight, and about how individuals often work *together* to cause failure. And we want to help you understand *why* we do these things to ourselves, even though we want so desperately to be slim and healthy.

JEFF: Right off the bat, I'm going to do what many of our esteemed leaders probably should have done, and that's begin with a full confession: I confess that I used to be a real idiot about the issue of weight. I used to think gaining weight was just a result of being lazy and undisciplined, and losing it was just a matter of willpower. I used to think all you had to do was eat right and exercise and you'd be slim—simple.

So back in 1980 when Norean began to gain weight shortly after we got married, I panicked. She didn't seem to know what to do about it, nor did she seem to *want* to do anything about it, so I took it upon myself to solve her problems for her. Talk about a big mistake! I pleaded. I whined. I coached. I criticized. I tried to get her to exercise. I hovered over her, watching her portion sizes and commenting on her junk-food snacking. I urged her to diet, because weight problems run in her family and I didn't want her to end up physically limited and unhealthy. When nothing worked, I got fed up and angry. Things went into the toilet, and we nearly flushed our marriage.

But, as they say, that was *then*. This is *now*.

Now I understand.

Somewhere along the way, I got smart. I decided there was more to this weight issue than just food and eating. So I threw off my preconceived notions and stereotypes and began to learn. I taught myself about the emotional complexity of overeating. Armed with new insight, I began to see overweight clients in group and individual therapy. I was able to help them in ways I could never help my own spouse. Then I began to realize my mistakes. It hit me how I'd been part of my wife's problems all those years. I recognized that the truth of the matter was that Norean's overeating wasn't the problem, it was a *symptom* of the problems both in her past and *in our marriage*. That's when things began to change.

NOREAN: I don't want it to sound like Jeff's to blame for all of this. It was a combination of a lot of issues—mine, his, ours. You see, I've had a long-standing emotional relationship with food. Back when we got married I weighed about 135 pounds. I'd kill to weigh that now, but at the time I felt fat. I had a lot of issues tied up with my eating. Food has always been a good friend to me. I ate for comfort. I ate for escape. I used my weight to protect me from closeness with others. I used it as a barrier to sexuality. I used my weight to express things I couldn't express any other way. I even used it to punish Jeff for things I thought he needed punishing for. So, because I ate for reasons that had nothing to do with my body's nutritional needs, I gradually gained weight, topping out at around 250 pounds after two children. On the surface I knew I didn't want to be fat, but underneath it all I wasn't emotionally ready to do anything about it. From time to time I tried to lose weight, but it didn't stay off. I tried every diet program under the sun and the only thing I lost was self-respect. I also tried several rounds of psychotherapy because I knew there was more to it than just what I ate. Jeff and I put our heads together trying to understand the complexity of emotional eating, and gradually the light began to dawn. It wasn't until I was able to recognize all of my emotional uses of food and the hidden payoffs of my weight—that is, until I was able to find and foil my fattitudes—that I was able to make a commitment to exercising and eating right. The solution came only after I found the courage to look inside myself and make sense of my chronic self-defeating behavior.

JEFF: We hope that by reading this book you'll be able to resolve your problems a lot more quickly than we did. Now, we'd like to tell you more about "fattitudes"—what they are, what they do, and how you can keep them from fouling up your weight management efforts.

ONE

■

FATTITUDES, FRUSTRATION, AND FAILURE

More than likely, you're reading this book because you're one of millions of people who suffer with a daily internal war.

You've probably struggled for years. You've tried all the diets. You've done the liquids, the pills, the grapefruits, the star-sponsored miracle plans. You've kept the food diaries; you've recorded your goals; you've put motivational pictures on the refrigerator. When you go through the checkout line at the grocery store, your eyes are drawn to the tabloids and magazines, all of which trumpet with each issue a new, effortless way to shed those pounds and get those tight buns, a sexy shape, and a washboard tummy.

You've given many weeks, and you haven't taken off the weight.

What's really frustrating is that you're regularly bewildered by your own behavior. You can't count the number of times when you've been on track, eating right, exercising, and lo and behold, you drop some pounds. Then you rejoice. You feel good. You're on the way. But then, something happens. Something throws you off course. The diet's not working anymore. In utter frustration, furious at yourself, you quit. Again.

So, you surrender. You stop doing many things you love to do and stop going places you love to go, since you dread running into people you haven't seen in a while. All because when you walk into a room, you *know* everyone is staring, everyone is judging, everyone is ridiculing. You don't play with the kids or grandkids like you want to, because you can't keep up with them. You know you should exercise, but you don't have the energy, so you sit around and hate yourself, asking the questions: *Why bother? What's the use?*

The strange thing is, you're capable and competent in most other respects. You work. You take care of the kids and the family. People turn to you during crises because you're "The Rock." You're

Supermom. Superdad. Maybe both. You're a perfectionist. Always trying to keep everyone happy. You're so good at helping others, but you can't help yourself.

You feel out of control of your eating—and out of control of your life.

So, you picked up *another* diet book. Is this one any different? We think so. We hope you'll think so, too. One thing you definitely won't find in these pages is a food plan. You won't find any menus, recipes, or fat gram tables. Because you don't need that. You know all that stuff already. Right? You could probably nail the nutritional analysis of any food set in front of you within seconds. Knowing *what* you should do is not the problem. What you *really* need is a new way to understand *why you don't do it*.

Fattitudes will provide that: a new way to look at and talk about an old problem, and a way to understand, once and for all, the universal obstacle to healthy weight management. This book shows you how to gain control by understanding your inner workings, and teaches you how to help yourself and quit hurting.

But, most importantly, it should help you recognize the hundreds of ways you destroy yourself and prevent your own success. You'll also be able to identify others who unwittingly help you along the road to failure. You'll learn how *not* to be your own worst enemy, which is what ties all overeaters together. It is the thread that connects everyone who struggles with weight, despite individual differences. *The universal obstacle to healthy weight management is self-defeating behavior.* And that's why we need to understand *fattitudes.*

WHAT'S A FATTITUDE?

Let's first understand how people work. The simplest way to put it is that we think, feel, and act. We don't sit around and let the world come to us; we're active creatures who try to make sense of things, who try to organize what we see, hear, and feel and make it all understandable. Generally speaking, we perceive, understand, and act in accordance with goals related to our personal well-being, psychological survival, self-esteem, and emotional comfort. A simple model of human behavior is that thinking influences both emotions and action. In that vein, a fattitude can be defined as *a thought, feeling, or pattern of thinking or feeling that leads to self-defeating behavior in weight management efforts.* A fattitude is a shorthand way of describing a complex psychological process that's often unconscious. What's really important to understand is that when fattitudes are afoot, failure follows; when you are prone to self-defeating behavior, *nothing* works—not even the best diet or exercise program.

A man or woman plagued by fattitudes is often an emotional wreck. There's an internal war of competing goals and motivations that produces what seems like an endless, tormenting conflict over staying on track with healthy living. A person with fattitudes usually feels preoccupied with food and dieting, has poor self- and body-esteem, and shows symptoms of emotional eating such as bingeing, grazing, and eating for reasons other than physical hunger.

You know very well what we mean. You want with all your heart to lose weight and to look and feel better, and you know what to do to accomplish this. But still you continue to do things that are counterproductive. You sabotage yourself just when things are going great. That's because you suffer from hidden fattitudes that exert a powerful influence over your decisions and behavior.

Fattitudes Result In . . .

- An internal war of competing goals and motivations
- Inner torment leading to emotional exhaustion
- Yo-yo dieting and weight management failure
- Shame, guilt
- Bingeing and/or grazing
- Preoccupation with food and dieting
- Poor self- and body-image
- Emotional eating

A fattitude isn't something you can observe on an X ray. It's not some gizmo in your brain that controls your behavior. A fattitude is a thought habit: an old, overlearned way of perceiving yourself and the world. Fattitudes may even be remnants of childhood survival strategies to which you still cling, operating automatically and requiring nothing deliberate on your part. They might be consistent, shadowy aspects of your mental outlook, or they might appear in momentary, imperceptible flashes of destructive energy.

Fattitudes

The best way to understand a fattitude is to put it into words. For example, Madeline was a fifty-year-old married woman who was fifty pounds overweight for about twenty years. She had tried all the diet programs without any lasting success, engaging in a frustrating cycle of losing and regaining weight for most of her adult life. She wanted to rid herself of her weight curse, but couldn't seem to sustain her efforts at healthy eating for longer than one or two weeks. She showed up at my office as a last resort.

As we worked together, we tried to look beyond what she ate and delve into why she ate. Little by little, the hidden conflicts became visible, and it became clear that Madeline was fighting a raging battle inside herself over the desire to lose weight. Although she wanted to slim down, there were opposing reasons why she needed to stay fat. Through self-investigation Madeline was able to identify and label ten specific fattitudes that acted as obstacles to her success. The most powerful of these had to do with her marriage, an unsatisfying relationship in which Madeline wished for romance and excitement, while her husband was content to sit around and watch TV. Madeline slowly became aware that one of her fears was that if she lost weight she'd become attractive again to other men. She feared she might not have the willpower to decline an extramarital affair, which might lead to the demise of her marriage, something she would find both frightening and morally unacceptable. Her primary fattitude: "I need my fat to save my marriage."

She discovered other fattitudes that were less prominent but still problematic, such as, "If I lose weight, people will expect more of me," and "If I get smaller, I might get 'run over' at work." Thus, Madeline had goals and motivations that competed with each other, and it was understandable now why she was unable to alter her lifestyle to lose weight: Her fattitudes got in the way.

Madeline's story is helpful because it illustrates the fact that fattitudes lurk and are often *hidden*. Madeline struggled for many years and had no idea whatsoever about the reasons why she failed. Fighting with fattitudes is a lot like boxing with the Invisible Woman or Man: You can't see the punch, but you sure can feel your jaw breaking. That's why insight is so important: If you can throw some paint on your unseen foe, you can jump out of the way next time he takes a swing at you.

Anybody can have fattitudes. They're not a result

of ignorance or stupidity. As one client, Danielle, thirty-five, wrote,

> *It was never a lack of knowledge that kept me from controlling my body size. I am a registered nurse. I went to school and learned all about the effects of nutrition on the body. Through my years of yo-yo dieting I became an expert on the latest weight-loss strategies. I know the significance of calories, fat grams, exercise, genetics—you name it. Knowledge does not necessarily ensure appropriate action.*

So, the message is that nobody is immune from fattitude infection, no matter how much you know about health, medicine, or even psychology.

The turmoil associated with hidden fattitudes is often intense and overwhelming. Many Fattitudes clients have entered counseling feeling exhausted and despairing of ever winning the battle. Sometimes they beat themselves up believing that weight management is really a simple problem with an easy solution. But overeating is a complex problem that's hard to solve, particularly when fattitudes are involved. One group member, Darla, forty-six, described it well:

It's not a food problem or a not knowing how to eat problem. It's about obsessing about food and being fat, and thinking that food is your number one problem in life. And that if you lost the weight and kept it off that you would be happy and your other problems wouldn't be so bad. It's about using food to shove down the anger, despair, hurt, disappointment, shame, humiliation, and feeling defective or not good enough. You give all you've got to others and don't get your own emotional needs met, and food is the only good thing you've got going for yourself all day long. You feel so empty inside and you just want to fill that empty space up. You keep trying to do it with food so you eat and eat until you're so full you can't think of anything else—except the despair of knowing you'll be gaining more weight.

It's *not* about food. Let's not forget that.

FATTITUDES AND INTIMATE RELATIONSHIPS

Intimate relationships can be considered the "baggage claim area" of life. We all know how painful and difficult close relationships are at times. If you ever want to measure someone's level of mental health, all you have to do is look at the quality of their involvement with others. Close relationships are the best theater for our emotional baggage to go on display.

The same goes for fattitudes. They come out to play most often when the issue of intimacy is stirred up. When we form or attempt to form a relationship deeper than mere acquaintanceship, the risks to our personal safety and psychological well-being sky-rocket. Remember the common kitchen-wall plaque? It says, "A true friend is one who knows all about you, yet loves you just the same." Often, we're afraid to be known for who we really are, since rejection hurts so much. When we let people into our hearts, we also face the risks of abandonment, loss, and psychological injury. So, when the stakes are high, as they are in intimate ties, our psychological survival strategies often kick into higher gear, and fattitudes become more troublesome and more plentiful.

By definition, a relationship requires two people. Which means, of course, not just one but *two* sets of emotional baggage with which to contend. The mix of personal problems and quirks can work out satisfactorily, if each partner is willing to look at his "luggage" and work at dealing with it. Or, it can create complicated snafus that derail the entire relationship. Fattitudes work the same way. There are many relationship patterns that act to create, maintain, and strengthen fattitudes and thus heighten the pull toward failure. When relationship fattitudes exist, the problem of healthy weight management becomes even more challenging to solve. Sometimes our failure is **assisted** by accomplices, people who inflict their own fattitudes on us. It is no wonder succeeding at weight loss is so difficult.

ONWARD AND UPWARD

Finding and foiling your fattitudes is hard, hard work. You didn't accumulate fattitudes overnight, nor will you rid yourself of them in that time frame. Lynn, forty-three, wrote, "The part of me that is an overeater has a strong, strong will. It's a daily effort and it can be exhausting and frustrating. But only I can do it for myself." And one of the best truisms to keep in mind is that *until you deal with the demons, you can't tackle the fat.*

So, that's where we head next. You've got to un-earth and identify your fattitudes, so you can end the frustrating cycle of self-defeat. In the next two chapters we'll discuss the two broad categories of self-defeating behavior: self-sabotage, when you fail completely on your own, and assisted sabotage, when you have an accomplice who works against your success just as hard—if not harder—than you do.

As the old proverb says, "A journey of a thousand miles begins with a single step." So read on! We've got a lot of work to do!

TWO

■

SELF-SABOTAGE:
HOW WE FAIL WITH
NO HELP AT ALL

One of my clients came to the office for a session about two months into our weekly schedule of psychotherapy, sat down, and looked at me as if something significant had just dawned on her. She said, "I've finally realized who's doing it." I waited a few moments for her to clarify, and when she didn't, I asked her what she meant. She said, "It's my father's voice. I hear him." Now, I knew this client wasn't hallucinating, so I assumed she was talking about the running dialogue of negative thinking in her head that we had spent so much time trying to understand. "He's the one who told you you'd never amount to anything?" I asked. She nodded, then began to cry.

We then talked about how she'd heard a never-ending stream of criticism during her childhood, a never-ending series of expectations she could never match, and a never-ending absence of true emotional support from either parent. "He's still in my head, telling me I can't be good at anything," she said. "He tells me I can't be successful, that I still don't measure up and shouldn't even bother trying. And the worst thing is, *I believe him.*"

Sometimes the authors of our fattitudes are from our pasts, voices we keep alive because they're so much a part of ourselves that we don't know what to do without them. Other times, the fattitudes come from more current sources. Whatever their origins, fattitudes lead us to fail at weight management. We have to identify the enemy before we can wage war against it. We can start by understanding the fattitudes underlying self-sabotage. They can be grouped into three categories: Diet Mentality Fattitudes, Fitness Fattitudes, and Feeling Fattitudes.

DIET MENTALITY FATTITUDES

In 1998, Americans spent close to $40 billion trying to get slim. Forty *billion* dollars. That's a whole lot of money. According to recent research, about ninety-five percent of those who diet fail, so that's a whole lot of money *poured down the drain*. Why do we throw away money on programs, pills, concoctions, equipment, and products that have this high a failure rate? Because the diet industry is clever, and employs a lot of very bright people who know how to market effectively. They spend a lot of money convincing *us* to spend a lot of money. And it's these clever marketing strategies that can be blamed for a whole set of fattitudes. We've been brainwashed and often we don't even realize it. We need to understand some of these toxic brain boogers in more detail.

"THERE'S A QUICK FIX OUT THERE SOMEWHERE, I JUST HAVEN'T FOUND IT YET."

Ahhhh, the quick fix. The magic bullet. The miracle pill. It's the holy grail of dieters everywhere. We search and search. We get excited by medical research that boosts our hopes about something coming down the pike that will cure this over-weight malady once and for all, without a lot of hard work. Just the other day I saw a news article that suggested in the next decade there will be a pill that can substitute for exercise in battling the decreasing loss of muscle mass that often comes with age. So, there it is again: We'll be able to sit around and get skinny—and fit.

The diet industry knows that's what we're really wishing. They *know* how desperate we all are for an easy solution. That's why they capitalize on our endless hope by presenting their products as quick, easy, and painless. Everywhere we look there's a new product trumpeted as the next cure. There's a new book telling us if we'd just eat this and not that, we'd lose weight. *Fast*. And, of course, we *buy* all of it.

Just take a short walk through the checkout line at the grocery store. Perfectly positioned where they know we stand, bored, looking for something to pass a few minutes, there they are: the tabloids, the magazines. Have you ever looked at the head-lines and compared them? They all say the same thing. They all use the key words that entice us into false expectations. One day I was doing a little informal research and wrote down the headlines on a cross section of women's and fitness magazines. Here's some of what I found:

Get fit the easy way

Easy steps to perfect fitness

Drop pounds for good—12 easy options

Burn holiday fat fast

Perfect hips, thighs, stomach, butt—fast

28 days to a knockout body

Simple secrets to instant willpower

Now, why do magazine editors plaster these headlines on the covers, and why do they publish articles with these titles? The answer, of course, is because they sell magazines. Again, we buy this stuff because we want it to be true.

Unfortunately, it's not.

The quick fix is merely an illusion. And if we get tied up in the illusion, it distracts us from the real truth, that successful weight management requires a long-term commitment to healthy eating and regular exercise. It's hard work. Nothing can change that fact. It's *very* disappointing to realize that there's no simple way out of our weight dilemma. If we give in to diet industry spin, we'll get distracted from our efforts to make permanent changes in the way we eat and live.

"I'M NOT LOSING WEIGHT FAST ENOUGH."

One of the nastiest pitfalls of a diet mentality is the npatience that it causes. After reading all those articles about rapid and easy weight loss, when we're on the right track and losing weight in a healthy manner (i.e., gradually, about a pound a week), we tend to feel like failures.

One of the most destructive habits that goes along with impatience is focusing on the scale and whether it goes up or down on a daily basis. We've equated weight with worth for so long that when the almighty scale doesn't plummet, our spirits do. This connection must be broken. Weight loss is not the only criteria by which we can judge success or health. Successful weight managers tend to avoid the scale—or even discard it—so they don't fall into the weight-worth trap.

Norean knows this quandary all too well. When she made her turn toward a healthy lifestyle and began to lose weight, I told her she'd be better off getting rid of our bathroom scale. She insisted that she needed the feedback to know she was on track with her goals. I let her go, not wanting to force anything on her. A few weeks later, she walked up to me and said, "Here," handing me the scale, "you do it." Quietly, the scale found its way onto a remote spot high atop a closet shelf.

"I HAD A BAD DAY; I MIGHT AS WELL QUIT."
Impatience leads to other fattitudes that cause us problems when we're dieting in a traditional manner. Traditional diets are synonymous with deprivation and frustration. We put food into "good" and "bad" categories, and the bad foods can become even more enticing once they've been forbidden. This black-and-white thinking leads us to be "on" or "off" a diet, with nothing in between. So, when we fall off the diet, it triggers a domino effect so that we think things like *I've blown it. I have no willpower. I'm never going to beat this.* This stream of thinking generally leads to *I'm no good. What's the use?* We throw in the towel and go back to square one, adding a few binges along the way.

There was an interesting study done a few years ago that compared the weight loss success of three different groups of people over the course of two years: diet only, diet & exercise, and exercise only.

27

After the first year, both the diet only and diet & exercise groups had lost a good deal of weight, and the exercise only group was a distant third. At the end of year two, however, there were some surprising results. The diet only and diet & exercise groups had both gained all their weight back, while the exercise only group had continued to lose weight gradually and keep it off. The results made sense for the diet only group, but what happened to the diet & exercise folks? The researchers concluded that a "diet mentality" causes such a counterproductive mind-set that if we encounter failure, we tend to quit our weight-loss efforts *across the board*. So, in the diet & exercise group, when the subjects ran into frustration, not only did they quit dieting, they tended to quit exercising as well.

Clearly, a diet mentality is destructive to healthy living. Black-and-white thinking only clouds our vision on the true path to success.

"AS SOON AS I LOSE THIS WEIGHT, I'LL BE ABLE TO EAT WHATEVER I WANT."

All we have to do is slap ourselves with a time-limited period of torture, get the weight off, then go back to our old ways of overeating and sitting around. But it doesn't work like that. A long-term problem like weight management can't be solved with a short-term effort. The diet industry doesn't tell us that though, for obvious reasons. Can you imagine an exercise machine that's promoted as "This is hard, sweaty work that you have to do four or five days a week, and you'll lose about three or four pounds a month, maybe. That is, if you don't quit." I doubt there'd be many takers.

If we don't change unhealthy weight-loss patterns, we will continue to fail. Here's a good rule of thumb: *Don't do anything on a diet you're not willing to do the rest of your life.* Following that guide will lead you away from tricky shortcuts and toward the lifestyle changes that are necessary. So, if you're not going to eat yogurt and salad at every meal forevermore, don't even start. You *know* you're not going to stick with it, and you'll only end up worse off than when you started.

"EVERYTHING WILL BE FINE IF I CAN JUST LOSE THIS WEIGHT."

Diet ads usually have upbeat, slender, gorgeous people in them. People without a care in the world, who don't have any of the stresses and hassles that the rest of us have. So, the implication is, if we'd just lose weight *too*, like *those* people did, we'd be happy campers. Such a trap! I've heard this fatti-tude so often in an initial consultation with a new client that it has become a warning sign of hidden troubles.

If we focus on food and weight as the problems, we get distracted from other issues that need atten-tion. In fact, that's one of the hidden payoffs of a diet mentality: As long as we're dealing with the diet, we have a focus, and as long as we have a focus, we don't have to look at emotional things that are painful.

Marla began therapy with this very fattitude, but gradually came to accept that she was avoiding *her-self* by adopting yo-yo dieting as a way of life. For many years, her dieting had been such a preoccupa-tion that she was able to ignore the unresolved grief from her mother's death, the trauma of being a child in an alcoholic home, and her exceedingly low self-esteem. She came to realize that she'd been sabotag-ing her weight-loss efforts for many years for a couple of reasons. First, she wasn't ready to confront the feelings of grief she knew were lurking inside. Second, even though she'd counted on losing weight as a panacea for so long, she also harbored the fear that it wouldn't *really* solve everything; it wouldn't *really* make her blissfully happy. "I couldn't face the disappointment of losing weight and not having the perfect life." Until she dealt with her unresolved pain and gave up her unrealistic fantasies, she was unable to commit to a healthy lifestyle.

A related fattitude is "I can't really be happy until I lose this weight." So many of us postpone doing things we enjoy, because we're too focused on the way we look. As long as we're overweight, nothing else matters. This becomes quite a trap. When we postpone our happiness we dig ourselves into a frustrating rut of dissatisfaction, and we don't nurture or treat ourselves with respect.

"I HAVE TO RELY ON SOME EXTERNAL SOLUTION BECAUSE I CAN'T DO IT ON MY OWN."

One of my Fattitudes clients was discussing his frustration with the major diet programs he had tried repeatedly over the years. So I brought up an interesting research study that demonstrated that eighty percent of subjects who lost and kept weight off had designed their *own* eating and exercise plans. In telling him this I wanted to emphasize the role of choice and control in healthy weight management. He looked at me and said, "But I can't count on myself to get the job done right."

His feeling was quickly confirmed by the others in the group, who all could attest to the underlying lack of self-sufficiency that drives the search for the magic bullet. Many overeaters feel so weak in the skills needed to navigate the potholes of life that they rely almost exclusively on finding someone or something outside themselves to solve the problem. This creates one of those nasty self-fulfilling prophecies. Looking for an external solution prevents the necessary development of *internal* coping skills, without these skills it is impossible to end weight management failure. A common statement among overweight individuals is, "I need policing from somebody else." They don't feel strong enough to achieve self-discipline. We'll talk more in Chapter Five about the FATS coping skills that are crucial for every weight manager to master.

"THIS WILL NEVER WORK."

A track record of failure is a common denominator of dieters everywhere. We've all failed. The vast majority of us have failed over and over again. Every time we approach a new weight-loss goal, we do so with failure in the backs of our minds. It's a truism in psychology that the best predictor of future behavior is past behavior, so when we approach dieting with an expectation that our current efforts will just be a miserable repeat of the past, we've just made a scientifically sound prediction. If we don't have faith in our efforts, we'll destroy them sooner or later.

One of my clients talked about the "diet sigh" that she'd come to know so intimately over the years. She'd tried hundreds of diets without any lasting success, and considered herself an expert on everything the diet industry had to offer. Her typical style was to approach each new effort with vim and vigor. She'd start her new diet on a Monday—which is, of course, the only day to start a diet—and then by Wednesday she would witness herself engaging in the early morning "diet sigh" as she thought about her latest weight-loss plan. The sigh was in anticipation of failure and was accompanied by the destructive fattitudes "Why bother? What's the use? This will never work." The "diet sigh" was the early-warning signal of surrender, because by Friday she was usually doing the "shoulder slump" of defeat. She, like most of us, bombed herself out of the water by letting failure fattitudes creep in and infect more hopeful thinking.

FITNESS FATTITUDES

We are a nation of sedentary citizens. Despite all the research that shows regular exercise is one of the best things we can do for ourselves, estimates show that seventy to eighty percent of us aren't physically active enough. We sit too much. We use remote controls too much. We let fitness fattitudes get in the way of developing healthy bodies. Here are a few of the more notorious ones.

"I DON'T HAVE TIME TO EXERCISE."

This is one of the most common of all excuses for not keeping physically fit: lack of time. Everybody's too busy, and the best of intentions gets shoved further toward the back burner.

A client was having a recurrence of his weight management difficulties. So I asked him how much exercise he'd been getting. He said, "I'm just too pressed right now. I've got the kids and their activities. I work forty hours a week. Then there's the household stuff. Last weekend I had to fix the crack in the garage floor and get the junk out of the attic. The basement had to be cleaned. The neighborhood watch committee was last night—" At which point I held up my hand and stopped him, saying, "Jim, you're not telling me about your time. You're telling me about your *priorities*." He sat in silence for a moment. Then I added, "You're just telling me all the things that are more important to you than your own health." It had an impact. He thought for a while longer, then said, "I guess I've never looked at it that way before."

Many of us don't look at it that way. We make time for all sorts of stuff, but we tend to neglect our own well-being. Time isn't the obstacle; *commitment* is. Norean and I both practice what we preach. We're busy professionals with two young children and a household to run, yet each of us finds enough time to work out at least five times per week. How? By making exercise a priority and setting aside time to get it done. Norean gets on the treadmill at 5:15 weekday mornings, and I get on when she's finished. In addition, she does strength training three days per week. Many things could interfere with this arrangement, but we don't let them. We find ways to maintain our exercise routines despite outside interference. And that's what you have to do.

"I GET ENOUGH EXERCISE DURING THE DAY."

Well, true, if you're an aerobics instructor. Many folks have strenuous jobs that help maintain muscle tone and burn calories, but most of us don't. Taking the stairs instead of the elevator is a great place to start, as is parking in the most distant row of the office lot. Unless your exertion is regular (three to five times per week), of sufficient duration (thirty to forty-five minutes), and of sufficient intensity (in your target heart rate zone), it won't be enough to result in healthy weight management and cardiovascular fitness. We should all avoid sedentary shortcuts when possible, but extra activity is key to success with weight. Although research suggests that even small increments in activity level can have a beneficial impact on health, if you want the best results, you have to sweat.

I had one client who worked in a major corporation that provided a state-of-the-art wellness and exercise facility for all employees. My client walked past the facility every day to get to his office. He felt very guilty for not taking advantage of the equipment, and tried repeatedly to plan spending his lunch hour working out. He always found something else to do that thwarted his fitness efforts, though.

We talked about his reasons for avoiding exercise, and he expressed fears about becoming out of breath. When I inquired about the nature of his anxiety, he began to explore it a bit more, and we ended up identifying that exercising and being "out of breath" brought him too close to unresolved feelings about his father's death from chronic emphysema. His father had lingered for months experiencing daily panic episodes when he couldn't catch his breath. After we identified and spent a number of sessions working through his grief, he was able to take advantage of the wellness facility. He then could truthfully say, "I get enough exercise during the day."

"I'm just too lazy."

We call ourselves all sorts of nasty names from time to time, especially if we're overweight. We all know being fat is a personal defect, right? This is a message sent throughout our culture. We're fat because we're dumb and lazy and don't take care of ourselves. It's understandable that overweight folks take these criticisms to heart. They become part of who we are. The real trouble starts when we act in accordance with these preconceived notions.

Shy people tend to behave in shy ways. Then

they get feedback from others which further supports the label of shyness, and simply confirms what the shy person already knew. The same thing happens for those who consider themselves lazy, or undisciplined. The label becomes a prison sentence. It gives us no freedom to change, and causes us to behave in self-confirming ways.

One of my clients ran into his self-applied label of laziness one day when I asked him when was the last time he'd done something a lazy person wouldn't do. He thought a few moments, then said, "Well, just yesterday I went the extra mile on a project at work. It was deadline time, and one of my team members had left something undone. So I scrambled to get the matter taken care of right. And we got the project in on time, and it got tons of praise from my V.P." Then I said, "So you're not lazy at work?" He said no. I asked, "You'll push yourself when it comes to pleasing somebody else, or when the situation demands it?" Again, he agreed. "So," I said, "you're only 'lazy' when it comes to your own health." He thought for a moment, then nodded. That was the beginning of his successful efforts at "deconstructing" his negative self-image and winning the battle with this fattitude.

"I'll Look Foolish."

Shame about our physical appearance can turn us into housebound phobics, which creates another major obstacle to exercising. Who wants to go to a health club and get on a treadmill next to a voluptuous vixen or studly muscleman? Who wants to get ogled like an alien? Not many of us. One of my clients loved taking walks around her neighborhood, but feared running into someone so much that she'd only walk after dark. She said, "They'll know I'm trying to lose weight. I just don't want anyone to notice me."

It's nice to have exercise equipment in our homes so we can exercise privately, but many enjoy the motivational boost of group activities. New exercise facilities are springing up that recognize this need among those not interested in flaunting themselves in the mirror as they sweat. Personal training programs are a good option, since many trainers work on a one-to-one basis in a more private setting.

If we get too focused on what we look like, though, we'll never take the necessary steps to getting healthier. I had one client who used a ski machine at her sister's house, but who also had a well-equipped Community Center just a short drive away. She would've much preferred the Center because of the weight and resistance training equipment, but she was too self-critical to risk exposing herself in such a public place. She was immobilized by her fears and resisted making even small changes in her unsatisfying existence. So, to give her a needed boost, a trip to the Community Center quickly became her homework assignment. With some gentle pressure behind her, she was able to get over the hump and soon found the Community Center to be a place she used to her great benefit.

"I'M SO FAR OUT OF SHAPE, I'LL NEVER GET BACK IN."

This is what I call Mt. Everest syndrome. If you're trying to get to the top of the mountain and focus your gaze at the peak, you don't see that the first step is what's important. If you don't take the first step, the others won't follow. Even if you've never exercised before, starting a moderate level of activity can have significant health benefits, regardless of your age. Studies have shown that individuals as old as seventy or seventy-five can increase strength, endurance, muscle mass, balance, and lung capacity by starting to exercise.

Exercise clearly helps prevent the aging process. The most important thing to remember is it's never too late to change—or to exercise.

"GOD SAVE ME FROM THIS TORTURE."

Who likes to exercise? I don't really enjoy sweating and feeling out of breath. But I do enjoy how I feel afterward, energized, like I've really done something good for myself. That's why I exercise. Back when I was in graduate school I played full-court basketball two or three times per week with some buddies and was in great shape. Lunchtime basketball didn't even count as exercise, it was fun. Nowadays I don't have a basketball court in my basement, so I have to make do with the treadmill, or "dreadmill," as one client called it.

It's been said that exercising is ninety percent mental, because if your head's not in gear, your body won't move. We can turn exercise into an arduous and dreaded task if we let the thought torpedoes sneak in on us. Have you ever watched the seconds tick down on the treadmill display and thought, *Is a second really that long?* It will feel like eons if your focus is on how much longer. *This is awful.* . . . If your thoughts are about the unpleasant sensations that accompany exertion, then you'll be less likely to do it again. Instead, focus on the numerous health benefits. Keep your mind centered on the end instead of the means, and exercise can be a much more appealing activity.

FEELING FATTITUDES

Emotional overeaters have a major problem with weight management because food is closely tied to emotional coping efforts. Thus, emotional eaters tend to eat for reasons other than physical hunger, which of course leads to excess calorie intake.

We're all emotional eaters to some extent. It's nearly impossible not to be, in a food-oriented society where eating is a part of celebrations and rituals—and a fundamental aspect of family life and interaction.

How much emotional eating is too much? Simply put, when it interferes with your health and happiness. On the next page is a quick self-test to see where you stand.

SELF-ASSESSMENT INVENTORY FOR EMOTIONAL OVEREATING

Circle the number for each item that best reflects your current lifestyle.

0=NEVER 1=RARELY 2=SOMETIMES 3=OFTEN 4=ALMOST ALWAYS

1. *I try, but fail, to lose weight and keep it off.*

   0   1   2   3   4

2. *I feel out of control of my eating.*

   0   1   2   3   4

3. *I eat when I'm not hungry.*

   0   1   2   3   4

4. *I turn to food when stressed or upset.*

   0   1   2   3   4

5. *I use food as a source of pleasure or reward.*

   0   1   2   3   4

6. *I think a lot about food.*

   0   1   2   3   4

7. *I can't seem to stay on track with weight management.*

   0   1   2   3   4

8. *I binge eat or graze.*

   0   1   2   3   4

9. *I feel ashamed of myself and of my eating.*

   0   1   2   3   4

10. *Food helps me deal with feelings.*

   0   1   2   3   4

TOTAL SCORE_____

INTERPRETATION:

0-10: NO OR LITTLE EMOTIONAL EATING: Your weight management efforts should be relatively uncomplicated by emotional issues.

11-20: MILD EMOTIONAL EATING: You may experience difficulty achieving weight management goals due to emotional obstacles.

21-30: MODERATE EMOTIONAL EATING: You will probably encounter emotional obstacles to healthy weight management and should consider counseling.

31-40: SEVERE EMOTIONAL EATING: Significant obstacles exist to healthy weight management, and counseling is strongly recommended.

Obviously, this is one test you'd be better off flunking. The higher the score, the more problems you'll probably have—and have already had—in your weight-loss attempts. Here are the most common and destructive feeling fattitudes that underlie emotional eating.

"FOOD IS FUN."

Well, of course it is. As stated earlier, food and eating typically take center stage in our entertainment activities. Our social lives are built around the act of consumption. We go out for lunch. Out for dinner. Out for drinks. We meet and greet friends over a plate of food. We never invite people over to our homes without giving significant thought to what we'll serve them when they're here. Ever try it? Call somebody and say, "Hey, why don't you come over for some . . . conversation? We're not going to have anything to eat or drink that might get in our way." More than likely you'd spend the evening by yourself.

Using food as fun isn't a problem unless it's the only fun you have, and you get into serving mouth hunger instead of stomach hunger. Mouth hunger has to do with all the nonphysical reasons you eat: It tastes good, it feels good, it's enjoyable to share this with someone, etc. Feeding mouth hunger almost always leads to overeating. Mouth hunger is hard to quench—very easy to trigger, and very hard to satisfy.

Another version of this fattitude is, "But I love to cook!" Well, okay. So what? Does leading a healthy lifestyle mean you can't have a good time in the kitchen? Of course not! Norean has always enjoyed cooking, and now has a great deal of fun finding ways to cook delicious food without relying on the old fatty ways she used in the past.

"Food is fun" is a fattitude that's probably present in just about all of us, although there *are* folks who just don't seem to invest much energy in the act of eating. They're usually slim and have a number of other satisfying hobbies that occupy their time. Children would probably develop in this manner if we didn't teach them so much about the emotional aspects of food.

"MY EATING IS OUT OF CONTROL."

The issue of control is usually central to the inner conflicts of the emotional overeater, and feeling out of control is a common subjective experience. The typical emotional overeater feels helpless and frustrated because of her history of failure at weight management. She usually feels as if she can't stop herself from overeating, despite knowing it's self-destructive. She often feels like her right hand is stuffing food into her mouth, while her left hand tries to slap it back onto the table.

Donuts don't really jump off the plate, and aliens don't invade our bodies and take over, even if it feels like they do. Eating requires the decision to eat. You are the only one who can initiate the action of putting food into your mouth. You are the only one who can control your eating. How to explain, then, the bewildering feeling of being out of control?

The issue of control makes sense if we understand that our decisions are influenced by both conscious and *unconscious* thoughts and feelings. Humans are complex beings. We can think one way and feel quite another. Many things we do occur outside our awareness, and our minds are driven by forces from the present *and* the past. So, it's entirely possible for a person to be consciously pursuing the goal of healthy eating while, at the same time, an unresolved, hidden issue influences behavior down the opposite path. Therein lies a paradox: One can feel completely *out* of control of eating while achieving the goal of staying *in control* by using food to solve an emotional dilemma.

Another reason we often feel our eating is "out of control" has to do with the psychological power of food. Food and eating become so closely associated with emotional things that they often substitute for experiences we can't get any other way. I've heard it said so many times that "Food never lets me down." It's so reliable, so dependable. If a creamy chocolate bar is what we want, we know where to get one. We know what it'll taste like. We know what it'll do for us. Food is so powerful, we often feel helpless to find anything that equals its emotional potency. And that leads us to feel out of control.

It's unfortunately too common that emotional eaters have had a number of life experiences in which they've felt out of control of things crucial to their safety, well-being, and self-image. Many have a history of sexual abuse, come from alcoholic families, or have suffered traumatic loss and abandonment. For these folks, food can be a primary source of comfort, mainly because it *is* such a controllable substance.

Brenda, a forty-year-old woman, had suffered sexual abuse at the hands of a sadistic grandfather and emotional neglect in her nuclear family. As a way of surviving, she grew up learning to please others and never learned a sense of her true self. She also never learned basic emotional coping strategies. When she was in psychotherapy she was often assaulted by intrusive flashbacks of episodes of sexual abuse, and one way she coped with these was to assure herself she had "more than enough" food in the house. She'd go to the grocery store and stock up on basic supplies, filling her pantry shelves until they were sufficiently "stuffed." She explained that food had always been the only dependable thing in her life, certainly more dependable than the people who were supposed to love and protect her, and food was the only thing that did not get obliterated by the traumatic reexperiencing of the abuse memories. "It's the only thing I can truly count on," she said repeatedly.

Associated with her use of food for self-sustenance was the paradoxical feeling of being out of control of her eating, which, again, arose from her feeling that food was the *only thing* that worked for her. She didn't know what else to do, but she also knew that overeating was destructive in the long run. Brenda worked very hard in therapy to develop basic trust and other coping skills so that her reliance on overeating gradually diminished.

We can see just how complicated the connection is between *eating* and *control*. If we let ourselves fall prey to the conclusion that we are out of control, we'll miss the important point that complex and hidden feelings can be acting upon our decisions. If we overlook the real bully, we'll never win the fight. One client talked about how he'd come to realize that his eating was clearly a result of a decision-making process. He said, "When I binge, I know it's my choice. Right now, I'm still choosing to do it, but at least I know *why*."

"I DON'T WANT TO FEEL, I WANT TO EAT."

One of my Fattitudes clients said exactly that one day about three weeks into her course of therapy, after she realized that her emotional life was the real source of her problems with food. "Can't I just lose weight and forget all this emotional crap?" she asked, in all seriousness. The answer, of course, is "no."

Underlying most emotional eaters' relationship with food is a significant weakness in handling feelings. They usually grow up in families where emotions are dealt with in inconsistent, chaotic, or neglectful ways. As a result, emotional eaters never learn basic emotional coping skills and thus often have to resort to less healthy techniques such as denial, avoidance, splitting off, or shutting down. The problem with these coping strategies is that they work only temporarily, leading to other costs later. A lifetime of avoiding feelings leaves something significant behind, usually, that something is a sense of self.

It's no wonder food has the emotional impact it has because it gets right down there into the stomach and provides a sense of being full. Food is unique. It helps squash feelings, something we call "stuffering" because it helps "stuff" our "suffering."

If our emotional life is something we've avoided for years, we tend not to understand our own feelings. We confuse emotional sensations like anxiety with hunger. Often, there's a frightening sense of something foreign lurking inside, and we become afraid to open the door, lest everything stuffed inside tumbles out into a giant mess. This is the dilemma that faces many emotional eaters when they come to the conclusion that they've got to confront their feelings if they ever expect to live a healthy lifestyle. Many go years avoiding such a conclusion. When they finally take the step to face things directly, it can be an overwhelming task.

Ruth feared that if she started crying, she'd never stop. Early in therapy she said, "Facing my feelings is like being in a life boat, alone, in the middle of a stormy ocean, like on a big roller coaster of waves." She feared she wouldn't be strong enough to handle all of it, but she was able to take small steps such as writing unsent letters to important people from her past. After one such letter to her mother, she cried profusely about her feelings of being overlooked and unloved as a child. In our next meeting, she talked about having lost a big chunk of her urges to binge, and we discussed how this was tied to her new courage to confront feelings she'd tried to hide from for so long.

"I NEED MY FAT BECAUSE _____."
One of the most pernicious of all fattitudes is when there are hidden payoffs to remaining overweight. Although it's easy to identify the downside of being fat, it's very common for overeaters to harbor unconscious reasons why they want to stay that way. This results in competing motivations, an internal war that pits the wish to be healthy against the need to stay fat. What follows then is the vexing start-stop-start-stop of yo-yo dieting.

The payoffs of pounds are plentiful. Fat can be emotional insulation, a barrier to intimacy, a protection against sexuality. It can be a way to feel powerful, or it can be a way to avoid recognition. As my client Margie said, "Being fat helps me feel invisible. Society tends to ignore me. And that's just what I want." It's true that overweight people tend to be disregarded, and many clients have said that they stay fat because people expect less of them.

Robert came into therapy wanting very much to lose a big chunk of his 285 pounds. As I always do in the first session, I asked him if he could identify any reasons why he might not want to slim down, reasons why he might want to remain overweight. He was bewildered, and looked at me as if I were insane. "Of course not," he said. "Why in the world would I want to look like this?" I dropped the matter, because it often takes some exploration to unearth the hidden payoffs.

Over the next few sessions, we worked on several issues, but one that came up repeatedly was that when he overate, he was preoccupied with the urge to get his "fair share" by eating quantities so large that he ended up almost immobilized. Things began to fit together as he talked about working in a family business with two older brothers who were very domineering. Robert slowly began to realize that his girth provided him a sense of power, in that he was literally "bigger" than his brothers.

He'd always felt shoved to the rear in his family because his brothers were both highly demanding. Robert had been an "accident" baby, born to older parents who really didn't have the time to raise an-

other child. Robert came to realize that a significant payoff for remaining fat was that it made it
more difficult, literally, for his family to "push him
away."

Identifying and resolving hidden payoffs is a key
to lasting weight management success. There are
times, however, that individuals come to realize
their payoffs and also realize that they're unwilling
to let them go. For example, after our initial session, Anne, a forty-four-year-old married woman,
decided not to pursue further counseling because
we talked about her eating having the payoff of
keeping her emotionally numb. She'd had a weight
problem for about ten years, following the breakup
of her extramarital affair. The loss had been devas-
tating. Her husband found out about the affair,
and after a period of separation, they eventually
were able to repair their marriage, even improving
it in some ways. The passion in her marriage had
never equaled the intensity of that with her former
lover, however. Losing weight required that she
come to terms with the feelings of loss she continued to avoid. Because she feared disrupting her
newfound marital stability, she concluded that it
was a can of worms better left unopened.

"IF I CHANGE, THINGS MIGHT CHANGE."

Basic fear of change underlies many overeaters' failure to take action against unhealthy living. Although the current situation may be unsatisfying, the unknown situation that would accompany change is even more frightening. Norean uses herself as a good example of this fattitude.

For years she'd used her weight as a barrier to sexuality and as a protection against being hurt. She'd considered changing many times and knew what it would take to be successful. Unconsciously, though, she struggled with what she'd have to face if she let go of her old ways of coping via eating. Changing might bring other changes she wasn't ready to face, such as feeling more vulnerable to others. She struggled with this inner conflict for many years, and it was only when her fear of what might happen if she didn't change (e.g., health problems, not keeping up with our children) became greater than the fear of what would happen if she *did* that she was able to commit to losing weight.

Marianne remarked one day during a group session that she'd been unhappy in her marriage for about twenty-five years. Several other group members said they understood, and the conversation turned to how lonely it felt in a hollow relationship. One member sat quietly through the discussion, and when I asked her what her silence was about, she said, "When Marianne talked about her marriage, my first impulse was to say to her, 'Why don't you just leave him?'" When I asked her why she'd held back, she said, "It struck me how empty my words would've been. I realized someone had asked me something similar about my job a few weeks ago. Why don't I just get a new job? If change were that easy, I'd have done it years ago."

One of the major reasons change is so difficult is because of our need to feel in control of the future. If we launch onto a new path, we have no way to reassure ourselves that everything will turn out okay, and that we'll be safe. Change is risky, but without it growth slows to a grinding halt.

Such was the case with Sam, who was married to a domineering and controlling woman. Sam usually said nothing about her rudeness, withdrawing into a resentful, angry mood during which he was prone to binge eating. Usually, the only time Sam ever spoke up about the relationship pattern was when he'd let his anger build up for so long he couldn't contain it anymore, which only made things worse. He recognized his need to learn to communicate in a more assertive and appropriate manner, but one of his biggest fears was that if he stood up for himself it might send his wife into one of her angry, depressive tailspins. And then things would only get worse.

We discussed at length how his wife had trained him to remain silent about his own needs, and how his neglect of himself was contributing to his overeating. A major stumbling block was Sam's fear that if he changed, things might change for the worse in his marriage. His fears turned out to be unfounded, and he was able to learn to set better limits in a diplomatic way. Once he began to behave more assertively, he reported being able to feel full on less food.

"IF I CAN'T BE PERFECT, WHY BOTHER?"

So many of us seem to feel that we have to be perfect in order to be acceptable. When inner feelings of inadequacy gnaw at us, we tend to see being perfect on the outside as a way to make up for what we feel on the inside. But, as we all know, perfection is unattainable. Perfectionistic behavior is a stressful way of life, because most perfectionists spend a lot of time feeling frustrated and disappointed with the way things turn out. The other danger with perfectionism that often plagues overeaters is rightly determining that being perfect is unrealistic, and then abandoning effort entirely.

Donna grew up with parents who inadvertently taught her that it was not okay to have needs of her own, and that the noble and worthy thing to do was to live her life in service to others. As an adult, Donna experienced a great deal of anxiety in trying to be the paragon of virtue expected by her parents. She found that she was never able to do enough to feel okay about herself. Guilt-ridden, Donna tried to fill herself up with food, which only served to further illustrate what an imperfect person she really was. At several points, Donna experienced emotional collapses, giving up on trying to be what she knew she couldn't be. While an inpatient in a mental health unit, Donna began to see that having needs and fulfilling them was a normal and healthy behavior, and that if she didn't take care of herself there would be nothing left to give to others. After outpatient therapy, Donna was able to abandon her perfectionistic goals and learn to live life as a regular person, not a saint.

**"I DON'T DESERVE TO BE SUCCESSFUL.
I DON'T DESERVE TO BE LOVED."**

This is the most fearsome fattitude of all. Most emotional eaters harbor significant self-esteem problems as a result of childhood neglect, emotional abandonment, and abuse. Often these feelings are strong enough that they result in an inner conviction of unworthiness, of being basically unlovable, or even of being "subhuman." When self-hatred is this intense, the consequence is behavior that is in line with this negative self-image. Those who lack self-respect make unhealthy decisions; people who hate themselves don't care what happens to their bodies. That's why we beat ourselves up and stuff our faces with food we know isn't good for us. For overweight persons, bingeing is a great way to inflict self-aimed anger.

When we experience failure on a consistent basis, we tend to develop an emotional intolerance to success, which often leads us to sabotage ourselves just when things are going well. Take, for example, Tricia, a nineteen-year-old college student from a blue-collar family. She had two older sisters, both overweight, and each got married shortly after graduating from high school. Tricia was a very bright young lady who had the capacity to do exceptional academic work, yet she found herself always teetering on the brink of a C average. She also lamented the fact that she was sixty pounds overweight and unable to attract a man. She wanted to do well in school, and she wanted to lose weight. But she had the nasty pattern of bingeing when she got upset, especially in the few days before an important exam. Not only did she gain weight, but she also got distracted enough from studying that she usually did poorly on her test.

It just didn't make any sense. Until, of course, she was able to understand that she grew up with a subtle but powerful pressure not to get "too big for your breeches" or too "uppity" because it made everyone, including her limited parents, feel ashamed and envious. Tricia unwittingly learned that it was safe to go only so far in life, because if she went *too* far, the perceived consequence would be rejection and abandonment by her family. Her pre-test binges were self-sabotaging but also self-preserving because they kept her from becoming too successful. Thankfully, Tricia was able to understand her hidden conflicts and take the steps to free herself from this self-destructive pattern.

Another client, Larry, forty-three, grew up with a depressed mother who spread her own misery; she hated when anyone else was happy. Larry was told repeatedly that he was no good and wouldn't amount to anything. Larry arrived in adulthood with a very fragile sense of self and limited confidence. He was very intelligent and talented, however, and got a job in a major corporation in which he rose through the ranks to a position of authority over a sizable team of employees. Despite his obvious talents, Larry was unable to truly accept credit for his accomplishments, and avoided relationships because he was certain he was unlovable. He worked intensively to identify his mother's negative messages, which had formed the emotional bedrock of Larry's self-identity, an identity contaminated with false and devaluing feelings and ideas. Larry lamented that he was "a middle-aged man who still cries 'Mommy doesn't love me.'" Larry was able to identify a related fattitude that he stated as "If I don't let myself hope, I can't be disappointed." Staying alone was safer than risking opening his heart to a woman to any significant depth, and it also kept him far enough from "life success" that he was able to tolerate his success in professional endeavors. Having a great job *and* a great family would've been too much for him to handle.

AND THE ENEMY IS US

We can go a lifetime in a pattern of self-defeating behavior and never have a clue about what's going on inside. Many dieters find themselves in this frustrating position. The good news, armed with insight into our fattitudes we can plan our attack strategy on the true foe. The bad news, sometimes we have to fight sabotage that comes not only from within ourselves but from without as well. That's our next stop.

THREE

■

ASSISTED SABOTAGE:
WITH FRIENDS LIKE THESE . . .

It's easy enough to fail at weight management, without someone else getting in our way. Unfortunately, there are often people in our lives who push us toward self-defeating behavior as our accomplices. Accomplices are those who act against our weight-loss efforts, who fertilize our fattitudes, and sometimes inflict their fattitudes on us. Accomplices can be anyone: spouse, father, mother, sibling, coworker, friend. Accomplices, like fattitudes, can act on us from the shadows, remaining hidden while they do their damage. They may not even be aware of their destructive impact on us.

How do you know if you've got a failure accomplice? Here's a list of "red flags" that usually show up in their behavior when you try to lose weight:

The Red Flags of Assisted Sabotage

- Change in attitude
- Withdrawal
- Criticism
- Denying importance of weight/health
- Erecting obstacles
- Food is more fun when you're dieting
- Overcontrolling
- Overinvolvement
- Premature publicity of weight goals
- "Pushing the buttons"
- General lack of support

There are plenty of ways to identify an accomplice. Anytime another's behavior gets in the way of striving toward success, there's a good chance their intentions are less than fully supportive. You go on a lower-fat diet, for instance, and suddenly your husband "rediscovers" the pleasure of dining out. You want to go to the gym, but your mother won't keep the kids for a few hours. Or, your wife comes downstairs to see you on the treadmill, and she says, "Well, I've finally gotten through to you, have I?"

RELATIONSHIP FATTITUDES

What can explain why someone would sabotage our efforts to be healthy? This seemingly irrational behavior can be explained by looking at *relationship fattitudes* that influence the behavior of those we rely on for support. A relationship fattitude, again, is a pattern of thinking or feeling *in someone else* that aids our self-defeating behavior.

"I NEED MY PARTNER TO BE FAT (AND DEPENDENT AND WEAK, ETC.) SO S/HE WON'T LEAVE ME."

One of the more common anxieties is the fear of rejection and abandonment. This concern has its roots in our being born utterly dependent upon others for our survival. As babies, we can't do anything for ourselves, and although we can grow up and learn to meet our own bodily needs, we still depend to a large extent on others for feelings of self-esteem and closeness. We fear being an outcast, because having social connections is one big measure of our success as human beings.

When we're in a relationship, or when we approach one, it's universal to have trepidation about whether we'll be judged adequate, or acceptable, and whether we'll be able to hang on to those we care about. Some of us avoid relationships entirely; others cling even when things are not going well.

There are a variety of ways we can ease our abandonment fears, some are healthy, like improving our self-esteem, and some are unhealthy, like doing anything to diminish the chances we will be left. If we fear abandonment, we feel less anxious if our partner has nowhere to go. And in our society, with its bias toward thinness, overweight persons can be seen as having fewer options because they're considered less desirable.

A classic tactic of the male batterer is consistent and systematic eroding of his wife's self-esteem, aimed at rendering her weak and dependent so he'll be less likely to be left alone. In other relationships the sabotaging strategies aren't as obvious or as brutal, but they are still powerful in producing the intended effects. For example, Andrea had been making a great deal of progress, losing about forty pounds and twenty-some inches over about a year's time by working with a personal trainer. Although much of her motivation came from the desire to look good in her wedding dress, she was also determined to remain healthy as a young wife and future mother. After she got married, though, things changed. She began to miss workout appointments. She began to make excuses. Her efforts trailed off. About two months after her marriage, she dropped out of the program. Calls to her home to determine what had happened led to her giving explanations, such as "I just don't have the time right now."

On closer inspection, however, it became clear that her new husband was overweight, and had been less than enthusiastic about her weight-loss success in the past. Andrea succumbed to her husband's fattitudes. He was secretly unsupportive of her efforts to slim down, because he feared he might not be able to hang on to her if she was so desirable. As she gained weight back, her husband became more relaxed, and illustrated a related fattitude, "If you stay overweight, I don't have to compete." Her husband felt less pressure to do something about his *own* weight problem if she shared the problem. Andrea's husband accomplished his sabotage in subtle ways, such as encouraging her to stay home instead of going to the gym, and communicating that he felt she looked fine the way she was. It worked to his benefit, but not to hers.

"I NEED A PERFECT PARTNER TO FEEL GOOD ABOUT ME."

This is a pattern that's in some ways opposite to the above, although it still has to do with self-esteem problems in the accomplice. When we have a feeling of insecurity or inadequacy, one way to pump ourselves up is to identify and associate with other people we see as ideal or perfect. We use our connection to such folks as a "medallion" of our own worth. The problem comes in when the "narcissistic extension" loses his or her glow of flawlessness. That's when the anxiety and fireworks occur. Sabotage in this scenario occurs as the accomplice becomes anxious, critical, and overinvolved in his partner's weight struggles.

Steve comes to mind as a good example of this situation. He'd struggled with his weight since leaving high school athletics and got married right out of college to a woman who was determined to climb the corporate ladder as quickly as possible.

Steve and his wife both had challenging careers, which required much politicking and job-related socializing. Events with his wife were an ordeal because of her pre-event "coaching" on what to say and not say, do and not do, and so on. And the after-event scolding for his missteps was an added torture. One of the things she picked on most was his physical appearance, telling him he was fat and needed to tone up, and that he was an embarrassment to her because of his weight. Unconsciously, Steve overate as a rebellion against feeling dominated. When he was able to identify his hidden feelings and express himself assertively, the quality of their marriage increased and Steve was able to make better choices about food.

"IF I KEEP YOU ONE-DOWN, I STAY ONE-UP."

One of the ego-boosting strategies we learn early in life, usually on the playground in elementary school, is that if we tear down somebody else we tend to feel elevated in comparison. Schoolyard bullies practice this technique with great frequency, to the terror and devastation of other kids. We need only look as far as our contemporary mudslinging political campaigns to see that this behavior persists into adulthood. It happens in marriages as well. For many, having a partner who is less successful is a neurotic way to feel better about oneself. Keeping that partner in a one-down position has a destructive payoff. Often, this pattern gets tied up with weight.

Sara had been married for about ten years and during that time had gained about sixty pounds. She entered psychotherapy against her husband's wishes because she was depressed and felt out of control of her eating. It became clear that marital issues were a significant part of her problems, so I suggested she talk with her husband about having some joint sessions to address what was going on. Of course, the husband refused to cooperate, stating that he didn't believe in psychology and didn't have any problems. Sara continued therapy and began to make progress in spite of her husband, who tried other ways to obstruct her efforts. He controlled the checkbook in the marriage, so when it came time to pay the therapy bill, I got used to waiting. Eventually, Sara became aware of the disturbing fact that her husband simply didn't want her to get better. Since he was unwilling to look at his own problems, Sara made the decision to pursue a divorce. Not the ideal outcome, of course, but when one partner is unwilling to change, working on marital issues is largely impossible.

"I'LL CONTROL YOU IF YOU CAN'T CONTROL YOURSELF."

As we said previously, control is a prominent issue for most overeaters, and is a source of much internal conflict. Often, this internal struggle over control can become *external* and can turn into a bone of contention in relationship power conflicts. When we get into a power struggle, the biggest problem is that someone has to win and someone has to lose. In power struggles there is no compromise, no middle ground, no easy give-and-take. Nobody wants to enter into battle just to lose the war! So, fights over food and eating can result in long-standing impasses that end up costing everybody involved a lot of aggravation, hurt, and in the end can prolong poor health.

One of the most common and difficult of all situations is when the struggle over food occurs between parent and child. I've witnessed this dilemma all too often with friends and clients alike. Mothers have come to me in a panic over their child's eating habits and weight gain. "What do I do?" they all ask, wanting to be supportive, helpful parents, yet not wanting their child to get fat and suffer the social ostracism that usually goes along with it. Often, parents try to set limits with the child's food intake, which usually amplifies the level of conflict. More often than not the child then begins to sneak eat.

I've also heard repeatedly from clients who grew up with intense scrutiny of their physical appearance, with parents who put them on diets at early ages and who thereby taught them that worth equals weight. It is usually the case that the power struggle over food turns into a struggle over feeling accepted and being able to express autonomy, and healthy weight management soon falls by the wayside.

The best solution to a power struggle is to not create one, and if there's already one raging, to defuse and refocus it. Parents in these situations need to back off and realize that the best way for their child to be healthy is for the child to adopt that goal by choice, not by having it thrust down his or her throat. It's disturbing, but true, that when we feel oppressed by someone controlling us we often choose the path of defiance to "win." We then remain autonomous, even when that means behaving in self-destructive ways.

Even long after the power struggles of childhood have passed, we can still struggle internally. The messages our parents transmit to us get implanted at deep levels, and we can carry on the battle even in the absence of a current enemy. Robin is a good example.

She grew up as an only child of overcontrolling and perfectionistic parents who clearly wanted their one and only offspring to be a prize in every way. Robin, although not objectively overweight as a child, was hovered over by her mother, and grew up feeling that every scrap of food she put in her mouth was subject to microscopic scrutiny. By age eight, she was hiding candy bars under her pillow at night, relishing in the forbidden pleasure of chocolate and gaining a sense of strength from her ability to defy her parents. By her teenage years, she began to gain weight, leaving her parents bewildered since they had watched her intake so closely. Then there were the multiple doctors' visits in search of some thyroid or metabolic problem that would cause such a weight anomaly, and when none was found, even stricter diets and exercise routines.

Needless to say, by the time Robin left for college she was about forty pounds overweight, and soon gained another fifty when she was free of the tyranny of her home and could eat whatever she wanted in whatever quantity. Her parents were devastated, and although they tried to maintain contact with her over the years, their continued embarrassment over her weight led Robin to move far away and see them only infrequently. She entered therapy because of her chronic low-level depression and feelings of inner emptiness, as well her compulsive eating. What we discovered was that Robin continued to express her "independence" by eating. It was only by unearthing this raging conflict and putting it to rest that Robin was able, for the first time in her life, to decide that her health was something *she* valued and that she wasn't "losing" by making peace with food.

"LET'S SQUELCH THIS SEXUAL PASSION BECAUSE IT'S TOO CLOSE FOR COMFORT."

How many times have you heard, or experienced yourself, that the quality and intensity of sexual relations tends to diminish after a couple gets married? It's all too common. During dating, it's all fireworks and explosions; post-wedding night, things get cold quickly. It's usually bewildering for the partners. For some, the combination of passion and commitment is a bit overwhelming, leading to feelings of being smothered and restricted. How this applies to sabotage of weight loss is that being overweight can be a "solution" to the sex-and-commitment problem, since for many couples fat creates insulation against intimacy and cools down the fire of sexuality.

John was a good example of this dilemma. John was twenty-seven years old when I first saw him. He'd been married for about four years and had gained weight steadily over that period of time. He told of his wife's frustration with his eating patterns, and that she'd done everything to try to get him to limit his portions and to work out. He attended the initial session with me only at his wife's prodding. Not surprisingly, he was reluctant to open up much in the first few visits, but we spent a good deal of time talking about the mutual dissatisfaction in the marriage, and his feeling that his wife was unable to accept him at his current weight. John did not want his wife to accompany him for couples work, instead preferring to figure things out for himself first. We talked about sexual matters and about how everything was just great while they were dating. Both found their physical relationship to be fulfilling, and John even remarked that his wife was quite "talented and lively" in bed. He related, however, that he recalled feeling something shift soon after they'd gotten married. They hadn't lived together before the wedding, so John had chalked his new discomfort up to the stress of moving into and maintaining a single household. He described feeling anxious and began to avoid physical closeness with his wife, and her frustrations were expressed in such a manner that all John heard was an increasing level of demands.

In response to the stress, John turned to food. It would've been easy to get distracted by the level of conflict that had intensified in the relationship, but to understand the root of the problem, I asked John to talk about what he'd felt after getting married that seemed to start it all. As he explored his thoughts and feelings, it became clear that John felt unprepared for the long-term commitment of marriage. He felt a lack of freedom and began to feel suffocated by the closeness with his wife, even though just weeks earlier their sex life had been spectacular. Further, John described feeling closed-in just like he had growing up with his over-protective mother.

John needed his weight to cement his autonomy by establishing a barrier around himself. We spent a number of sessions helping him work through this internal conflict so he could make a more satisfactory adjustment to marital intimacy and, eventually, effective weight management.

"LET'S FOCUS ON YOUR PROBLEMS SO I DON'T HAVE TO LOOK AT MINE."

Just like a lifetime of dieting can distract us from other painful problems, in some relationships there's a payoff for having one partner occupy the "sick" role. This happens frequently in families with a "problem child" who is unmanageable for unknown reasons—until it becomes apparent that both parents need the child's misbehavior to help them avoid looking at a deeply distressed marriage. When this situation is present, both parents unconsciously promote the child's difficulties and resist efforts to solve them, since the result would be the unearthing of something more uncomfortable. The same thing is true with overeating. Being overweight is enough of an "illness" in our society that in a marriage it can be a convenient focus for both partners.

Don and Terri had been married for nine years. Don had a significant weight problem, having gained almost a hundred pounds since their wedding day. Don's weight was causing considerable distress in the marriage, and their sex life had been pretty much nonexistent for the majority of their time together. We worked diligently in marital and individual therapy, addressing Don's issues from his alcoholic family of origin, and began to make progress with his move in the direction of healthy eating.

It was usually the case that when Don began to lose weight, the other conflicts in the marriage would intensify. After several repetitions of this pattern, I called attention to the fact that Don's progress seemed to get derailed each time he got on the right track, and I suspected some hidden payoff for his being "sick." I asked them what possible benefit did either or both of them get from Don being fat. Although each initially drew a blank and scoffed at the idea, reluctantly, Terri was able to explore her feelings about the sexual discomfort she'd felt early on in the marriage, and with further nudging was able to admit that sex made her anxious. Terri had a history of sexual abuse that she'd never faced, and Don's weight gain (and the resulting absence of sex in the marriage) provided a convenient way for her to continue to avoid the pain from her own trauma.

"I DON'T WANT TO MAKE MY CRITICS HAPPY."

Another way power struggles show up in relationships has to do with the big issue of "Can you love me for who I am?" Because our society places so much emphasis on slenderness, overweight folks have to deal with ridicule and criticism from just about every direction. One of my group clients said, "You know, criminals, liars, sex fiends, alcoholics, they can all walk around in public and nobody knows a thing. They can put on a reasonable impression of being a normal human. Me, I *wear* my problems. Everybody can take *one look* and see that I'm all messed up inside. It's not fair, being so transparent."

Most overweight people feel a lot of anger at being judged, which tends to complicate the decision to lose weight. Remember the old saying, "If you can't beat 'em, join 'em"? For people plagued with weight problems, the saying becomes "If you can't beat 'em, beat 'em harder, then beat yourself."

Because, what happens when we lose weight? We become pleasing to others! Those bastards that put us down all the time, now they're telling us how *good* we look! It's quite a quandary, making someone happy who has made *us* so *unhappy* for so long.

When a woman begins losing weight the situation is often very delicate socially. Most people make the mistake of praising her, saying things like "Have you lost weight?" or "You're looking great!" On the surface, these are compliments. But to the formerly overweight woman, the comments are often enraging. Why pay attention to me now? Where were you when I was fat? If you think I look great *now*, you must've thought I looked *terrible* before! I've worked with many clients who begin to sabotage themselves just when people begin to notice their progress.

Barb had an elderly mother who was a weight fanatic. Whenever Barb risked visiting home, she was always subjected to a "tummy surveillance" for recent weight gains or losses. More often than not, Barb would hear lectures about eating and low-fat diets and health risks of obesity and *this is what works for me, honey*. The visits were so unpleasant that Barb found every excuse not to stop in. Once, after about a month's time in which she had only telephone contact, Barb stopped in, having lost about four or five pounds via exercise. To her surprise, the visit was even more unpleasant than all the others because her mother was *praising* her for doing such a fine job with her eating! It was so uncomfortable that Barb bolted from the house and talked in her next session about having binged on ice cream immediately after leaving her mother's presence.

"THE FAMILY THAT EATS TOGETHER STAYS TOGETHER."

We know that overweight tends to run in families and thus has certain genetic roots. In many families, though, being overweight is part of their feeling of "togetherness." When that's the case, sometimes it's very hard to break the mold, and family members might even react negatively to one of the brood striking out in a new direction. Losing weight in such a family might result in emotional consequences that get in the way of continued success.

Rick was thirty-five years old and divorced when he came to see me. He'd struggled with his weight for most of his adult life. His mother was overweight, as were both of his older brothers and his younger sister. The atmosphere in the family was one of "we can't fight it, so let's revel in it." His mother was a great meat-and-potatoes cook who enjoyed putting out lavish spreads of high-fat food, and attendance at Sunday evening dinner was an assumed commitment.

Rick felt a strong tug not to do anything about his weight. He never felt comfortable discussing his concerns about his health, or the health of his parents and siblings, because the "family close-ness" expectation was too set-in-stone and invio-late. He struggled with the fear that if he began to eat right, exercise, and then lost weight, he'd soon face something akin to shunning. He believed that his parents were very insecure individuals who needed the "discipleship" of their children in order to maintain adequate self-esteem. His attempts to discuss his concerns openly with his family met with stunned silence. So, Rick had a tough deci-sion to make.

We worked a long time on building his self-confidence and his belief that he could stand on his own two feet, since independence training hadn't really been emphasized in his family. In fact, Rick pointed to his overdependent relationship with his wife as the major cause for their divorce. Only when Rick became more self-sufficient was he able to begin his trek toward health. And although reluctant to accept it at first, his family came to believe that their allegiance didn't necessarily depend on a shared body type or group consensus that health was unimportant.

"YOUR SUCCESS IS MY SHAME."

A related fattitude has to do with the impact of your weight loss on friends and loved ones, particularly when being overweight is part of the bond. Misery loves company, and when the company's no longer as miserable, it tends to shake up the balance. In many such relationships, there is often the unstated pressure to remain in an unsuccessful life position because the connection couldn't survive otherwise. I had one client who found herself in this very predicament.

Liz had been overweight for about twenty-five years and had a clear track record of yo-yo dieting due to some significant problems with emotional overeating. She worked in a large company and had become close friends with a coworker, another woman with weight struggles. Their friendship was primarily work-related, although occasionally they socialized in the off hours. They'd become diet buddies. Over the years they went on numerous diets together, lamenting the deprivation, applauding their joint successes, and then crying over their joint failures. They usually ate lunch together, and Liz had grown to deeply appreciate her friend's support.

At one point, Liz decided to enter therapy, but couldn't convince her friend that it was a good idea. Her friend just wasn't ready to take such a step, so Liz decided to try it alone. She made very good progress in identifying her fattitudes and, as a result, began to exercise and to gradually drop weight. When this occurred, Liz ran into the obstacle created by her work friend: The friend was clearly upset about Liz's progress, although she tried to be a supportive cheerleader. The friend didn't speak of it directly, but gave the impression she felt left behind.

Liz was hurt by the change in their relationship, and was temporarily thrown off track. When she realized her friend seemed pleased that Liz was once again in a failure mode, she was able to resume her healthy lifestyle despite the fear she'd lose a friend in the process. Sure enough, as Liz lost weight the lunchtime commiserating began to decrease in frequency, and Liz had to confront the issue directly with her friend. Although it helped, the relationship was never the same, and Liz had to move on to others who could be more genuinely concerned with her success and well-being.

It's true that when you change, other aspects of your life also change. Your weight management success can result in changes to your relationships that might be very difficult.

So, What Do We Do About It?

Now that we've discussed all the reasons why weight management is such a problem, it may seem like an even more formidable challenge. So we need a good plan to battle these destructive fat-titudes. That plan involves a new way of looking at dieting—and a new way of understanding the word diet. Let's learn how to DIET our way to fattitude freedom.

PART II

•

FIGHTING YOUR FATTITUDES: THE FATTITUDES DIET

FOUR

■

"D" IS FOR *DISCOVER*

To end your long-standing history of weight management failure, to beat your cycle of self-defeat, to finally reach the pinnacle of personal success, we're going to tell you to DIET. We must be out of our minds. Right? Wrong. This isn't an old diet. This is a *new* DIET.

The next part of the book provides a four-stage self-help program aimed at finding, fighting, and foiling your fattitudes. Here you will learn to be your own best friend instead of your own worst enemy, by building awareness and self-understanding that eventually will lead to new, healthy behavior. It's not easy. It's not a quick fix. It's a process that is often quite painful.

LET'S TALK ABOUT CHANGE

If change was easy and straightforward, there'd be no need for counselors, psychologists, or self-help books. If it was easy to be different, who among us would choose to stay the same? Not many, I would guess. We'd all be happy, we'd all feel good about ourselves, we'd all have good relationships, and we'd all probably be slim and trim. Unfortunately, life isn't set up that way. Life is difficult and change is even more difficult.

WHY IS CHANGE SO DIFFICULT?

I had a client once who wanted desperately to end her cycle of self-defeating behavior and depression, but had never been able to find the key to making progress. She said one day in session, "I'm so fed up with being too much of not enough." She was frightened of taking any steps toward success. She'd been in the "failure" role for so long that it was second nature to her, and she didn't know how to act like a success.

Sometimes we don't change because we're scared to do so. Other times, we're not sure *how* to change, or what to do. As the fattitude says, "If I change, things might change." And if things change, we wonder if we'll be able to handle the new challenges and stresses of stretching ourselves beyond the unsatisfying status quo. What will people expect of me, if I risk moving forward? Will I be able to meet all the new demands? Will I have success, then only have it taken away? Isn't it better not to hope for things, because hope is dangerous?

One of my clients expressed her apprehension about the path ahead by writing the following poem:

FEAR
(BY ANONYMOUS)

I look at tomorrow with fear in my heart,
Uncertain this path I'm preparing to start.
Can I change, can I learn, can I truly succeed,
This hunger inside me to finally feed?

This fear runs so deep it's a bottomless pit,
It seems like a darkness that cannot be lit!
These mem'ries and heartaches, I fear I can't cope,
So what if I start and then find there's no hope?

This fear, this fear, it's a tangible thing,
Fear of the past and what tomorrow may bring.
It crushes my heart, brings gray clouds to my mind;
Am I able to face these monsters I'll find?

And what if it's me, this dark demon inside?
Who will I be if I no longer hide?
If I fin'ly stop running, who will I see?
A devil with fangs, or a lovable me?

Such is the anxiety associated with self-discovery, particularly if we have a history of denial and avoidance.

Another thing that makes change difficult is that humans are creatures of habit. We get into automatic patterns of behaving, often not even thinking about why we do things. Personality could then be defined as everything about which we say, "That's just the way I am." Perfectionists don't have to wake up in the morning and decide, "I'm going to be a perfectionist today." They just *are*. They pursue perfection just as a knee jerks to a physician's rubber hammer. To do things differently, we have to make an energetic effort that at the outset often seems impossible.

What can we do to disable our inertia? What

does it take to get better, to take a different path, to create a new way of living?

THE INGREDIENTS OF CHANGE

First and foremost, change requires three types of motivation: energy, readiness, and willingness. We have to put forth the effort, because changing takes a lot of hard work. We also have to be in enough discomfort and pain over our current patterns to feel ready for something different, even if that means taking risks. We also need to be willing to accept change and everything that follows from it, because a change in our behavior will send ripples through our lives and our personal networks. If these motivations don't exist, efforts at change will be frustrating and probably unsuccessful.

Second, to change we need to learn. Not just intellectual learning, but also emotional learning. We need information. We need to be taught about the obstacles we've created and to be educated about new ways of doing things we haven't tried before. We need to learn why we've made the mistakes we've made all along. That's what self-help books are all about. We're supposed to learn something that we can put to good use in our lives.

Finally, we need support. The number-one factor

in permanent lifestyle change is having some form of social group or peer network to function as cheerleaders and change-buddies. Recent research shows that social support more than doubles the chances for long-term weight management success. We need people to help us down the road to something new, whether that be a friend, spouse, partner, support group member, or therapist. Unfortunately, as we discussed in the last chapter, many times the people closest to us *resist* our efforts to change, because they, too, have gotten used to us behaving in certain ways and may not be ready for us to be different. Again, when *you* change, *things* change, and the people around you might have to change, too.

SELF-HELP TOOLS

The Fattitudes DIET program is based on an underlying process that can be expressed as

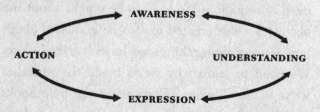

These four factors overlap and are mutually reinforcing and interactive. We need to learn about ourselves and the obstacles we've created. We need to understand how to do things differently. We need to express our feelings so that old baggage and issues can be resolved to allow us to move forward. And finally, we must translate our new knowledge into action that helps us achieve success. If one part of this process is left out or de-emphasized, efforts at change will probably fail.

As anyone with any "fix-it" experience whatsoever can tell us, there's nothing quite like having the right tool for the job. Nothing makes a task easier than having that socket wrench that really fits. Nothing makes a job more frustrating than trying to tinker with a tool that's inadequate or misapplied. So what are our tools for finding, fighting, and foiling our fattitudes?

Self-Help Tools
- Information gathering
- Self-expression
- Sharing
- Daily activities
- Goal setting
- Structured challenges
- Self-reward

We'll use all of these tools in the Fattitudes DIET.

Now, before we get started, a word about DIET-ing. Some of you may be put off by our choice of DIET as an acronym for this approach. Dieting has such a negative connotation, and it's been a source of pain and frustration for so many of us, why choose to perpetuate the label?

The answer is because the word diet is such an automatic part of our vocabulary. It's our goal to give it a new level of respectability by taking it apart and putting it back together again—the right way. To rid ourselves of our outdated and ineffective notions about losing weight, we need to destroy the old diet, since it has become such a nasty word.

PHASE ONE: *DISCOVER*

Phase One of the DIET requires that we **Discover** our feelings, thoughts, unresolved issues, and most important, our fattitudes. We have to understand why we fail before we can succeed. We have to know what we're up against before we can take proper action. So, we need to look inside. We must defocus from food and look at what's beneath our lifestyle and eating decisions, and we have to understand the connection between food and feelings.

For many overeaters, this is an unnatural act. Overeaters generally aren't primed and ready to take a look inside, because overeating is usually aimed at hiding the truth. Overeaters live their lives in self-protective ignorance for so long that stopping and facing directly what lies inside is a terrifying change. But it's also a necessary step.

Often, what makes facing feelings so difficult is needing to face what first caused the feelings. Confronting issues from the past that have contributed to adult ways of being means looking the demons in the eye so they'll back down and go away. Most fear that if they look at these internal demons something worse will occur. The hurt will worsen and they will have stirred up more trouble than they can handle. They'll end up weak and shamed. But it's only by having the courage to look at problems and issues squarely that we can convince ourselves we're up to the task of getting better.

TUNING IN

Let's start out by getting to know you. Take a look at the Fattitudes Sentence Completion Form and fill it out. Just write the first thing that comes to your mind, and try to be honest with yourself. There aren't any right or wrong answers.

Fattitudes

SENTENCE COMPLETION FORM

1. My name is _____.

2. My age is _____.

3. My weight is _____.

4. My height is _____.

5. My goal weight is _____.

6. I can describe myself as _____
   _____.

7. The thing I like best about myself is ____.

8. People who know me say I'm _____.

9. The thing I like least about myself is ____
   _____.

10. My biggest weakness is _____
    _____.

11. My biggest strength is _____.

12. One of my biggest fears is _____
    _____.

13. I worry too much about _____.

14. One of the biggest joys in my life is ____.

15. I need _____.

16. I want _____.

17. People hurt me by _____.

18. I am my own worst enemy when I _____.

19. When I eat, I feel _____.

20. Dieting _____.

21. I deserve _____.

22. My job _____.

23. One of my biggest stresses right now is ____

    _____.

24. One of my biggest satisfactions right now is

    _____.

25. What holds me back is _____

    _____.

26. Everything would be okay if _____.

27. People _____.

28. My childhood was _____.

29. Food _____.

30. I can never seem to _____.

31. One thing I've always wanted is _____.

32. It hurts when _____.

33. The person whom I trust the most is ____.

34. The person who has hurt me the most is ___
_____.

35. My biggest obstacle is _____.

36. I need my fat because _____.

37. The thought of being slim _____.

38. It scares me to think about _____.

39. I feel good about _____.

40. In the future _____.

41. Things I feel proud of are _____.

42. I admire _____.

43. What nobody realizes about me is _____
_____.

44. What scares me about changing is _____
_____.

45. I need _____.

46. I really need _____.

47. My fat protects me from _____.

48. The way I defeat myself is _____
_____.

49. My needs _____.

50. What bothers me the most is _____

_____.

51. If I could change one thing it would be __

_____.

52. What I remember most about growing up
    is _____.

53. My past _____.

54. I believe _____.

55. What nobody knows I need is _____.

56. If someone only knew _____.

57. When I see an overweight person _____

_____.

58. Losing weight scares me because _____.

59. I'll know I'm getting better when _____.

60. What I really want is _____.

Look over your answers. Did you learn anything
new? Did you have trouble answering some items?
Which ones? Which ones were easiest to complete? Which ones brought the most feelings to the
surface?

If you're like most overeaters, the negative sentence fragments were easier to complete than the positive ones. Self-critical thinking is automatic; it's a lot harder to find the good things about yourself or your life. By the time you're done reading this book, I hope that will no longer be the case.

The purpose of the Sentence Completion Form is just to get you to tune-in to yourself. You can refer back to it from time to time, particularly to see how your answers may change as you progress.

FINDING YOUR FATTITUDES

Next, zero in on your own fattitudes. This is a crucial first step in ending your cycle of self-defeating behavior. You may already have a good idea of the fattitudes that plague you. As a clarifying activity, though, fill out the survey that follows and see where you stand.

"D" Is for *Discover*
Fattitudes Finder Form

Rate your degree of agreement with each of the
following by using the scale below.

1 = Disagree Strongly 2 = Disagree Moderately
3 = Disagree Mildly 4 = Neutral, Not Sure
5 = Agree Mildly 6 = Agree Moderately
7 = Agree Strongly

1. I always look for the quick fix. _____

2. As soon as I lose my weight, I'll be able to eat whatever I want. _____

3. When I try to lose weight, it never comes off fast enough. _____

4. I have to rely on some external solution because I can't do it on my own. _____

5. When I have a "bad day" on a diet, I might as well quit. _____

6. Everything will be fine if I can just lose this weight. _____

7. Trying to lose weight never works. _____

8. I don't have time to exercise. _____

9. I don't like to exercise because I look foolish. _____

10. Exercise is true torture. _____

11. I'm so far out of shape, I'll never get back in. _____

12. I hate to sweat. _____

13. Food is too much fun. _____

14. My eating is out of control. _____

15. Food is my only reward. _____

16. Food helps me stuff my feelings. _____

17. There are reasons why I want to stay overweight. _____

18. I can't be happy until I lose my weight. _____

19. If I can't be perfect, why bother? _____

20. If I take care of myself, I'll be selfish. _____

21. I don't deserve to be successful. _____

22. I don't deserve to be loved. _____

Each of these items illustrates a specific fattitude that we've found common among overeaters. Which ones really strike a chord for you? Those items you score highest on indicate your most problematic fattitudes. Add up your score. The higher you score, the more fattitudes with which you have to contend.

The Fattitudes Finder Form is not complete. You

may have identified other fattitudes that we have not mentioned. What are your personal fattitudes?

Next, create a written list of all the fattitudes that get in the way of your weight management efforts. Write them down as "I" statements (e.g., "I need my fat because it's an excuse for failure"). Write down every fattitude that fits your particular situation. It's very important to create as complete and as specific a list as you can. Once you've completed your initial effort at this task, set the list aside, but add to it whenever something hits you and you can identify another fattitude. This will turn out to be a "cognitive map" that will help you identify what you're up against. We'll talk more about how to plan your fattitude-attack strategy later. Right now, just focus on finding as many of them as you can. You can use the following form to organize your efforts.

ILLUMINATING THE PAYOFFS OF POUNDS

Have you already identified the hidden reasons you want to stay overweight? Have you been able to determine what it is about losing weight that makes you uncomfortable? Do you have a partial idea that needs fleshing out?

Help yourself unearth these payoffs by closing

your eyes and imagining yourself in the near future, having lost the weight you want to lose. What would you be like? What would you feel? How would things change? How would your relationships be different? If you feel twinges of anxiety, you're onto something. Ask yourself why you feel scared about the image of being thinner. What's your inner conflict about losing weight? What will you lose in *addition to* the extra pounds?

Challenge your thinking in this regard by completing the following Internal Debate Form.

"D" Is for DISCOVER
MY FATTITUDES FORM

These are my personal fattitudes. These are the thoughts, ideas, and feelings that lead me to defeat my efforts at weight management.

_____

_____

_____

_____

_____

_____

_____

_____

_____

_____

_____

_____

_____

_____

_____

_____

_____

_____

_____

_____

_____

_____

Fattitudes
INTERNAL DEBATE FORM

I want to lose weight because	I want to stay overweight because

Almost all overeaters who repeatedly fail at weight loss engage in an internal debate every day. The problem in putting words to it is that the debate often is unconscious. We don't realize we're struggling with two opposite poles of an intense argument, but our self-defeating behavior gives us the evidence. So, writing down the internal debate is a tough task. It's also usually eye-opening, because many have never thought about the *benefits* of carrying excess weight. But the payoffs are usually there. The magnitude of each payoff is what's crucial to discern. The more significant the payoff, the bigger the obstacle to getting healthy.

Right now, you're just identifying the payoffs. We'll talk more later about what to do about them.

Another helpful exercise would be to make a list of each specific payoff you can identify. Ask yourself, why do I want to remain overweight? Why do I need my size? What does my fat do for me? Don't let yourself get away with answering "nothing." You can give some order to your payoff list by using the sheet on on page 108.

THE FOOD-FEELINGS LOG
Another tuning-in technique is to begin keeping a daily record of your food intake. You've proba-

Fattitudes
MY PAYOFFS FORM

These are my specific payoffs for remaining overweight:

_____

_____

_____

_____

_____

_____

_____

_____

_____

_____

_____

_____

_____

_____

_____

_____

_____

_____

_____

_____

bly done something like this before, measuring food and counting calories and fat grams. This log is a bit different. We're not interested so much in what you eat or how much, but more in what you *feel* before, during, and after you eat—particularly when you find yourself eating for no apparent physical reason.

You need to find your triggers and your personal connections between food and feelings. You need to open your eyes to your personal truth about food. You can then unearth the hidden issues that are driving your decision to use food in your emotional coping efforts.

It doesn't matter what format you use, but we've supplied a sample of the structure your Food-Feelings Log might take.

Begin keeping the Food-Feelings Log on a daily basis. You'll use it in the Fattitudes Focus Session discussed a little later.

JOURNALING

Another excellent tool for self-expression and discovery is to keep a daily journal. A journal can be a private place to express your innermost thoughts and feelings, a place to get some perspective on what you think and feel, and a place to identify issues that might be in your way. It's also a great way to keep track of yourself as you embark upon a journey of self-discovery and change. Progress often takes place in bits and pieces of insight, and it's helpful to document things in your journal so that in looking back you can understand changes that have taken place. A journal can also be a good way to reward yourself for taking positive steps.

A suggested format for journal writing is shown on page 112, but feel free to use any format you find helpful.

The purpose of keeping a journal is to express your innermost thoughts and feelings. Try to write from your gut rather than your head, and don't concern yourself with irrelevant things like neatness, spelling, sentence structure, etc. This is for *your eyes only,* so let it be a tool for your complete and honest disclosure. What are you feeling? What are you thinking? What did you *really* want to say to your boss today? Don't hold things back.

FINDING SABOTEURS

After reading Chapter Three on assisted sabotage, you probably have a good idea whether or

"D" Is for DISCOVER
FOOD-FEELINGS LOG

DATE _____

Ate When? Ate What? Ate Where? Felt What?

_____

_____

_____

_____

_____

_____

_____

_____

_____

_____

_____

_____

_____

_____

_____

_____

_____

DATE _____

Today I felt

The problems and difficulties I ran into were

I was pleased with how I

I need to work more on

Tomorrow my goal is to

not you're plagued by a saboteur. Can you identify one? Several? Are they aware of their impact on you? What are their strategies for aiding your self-defeat? Are the strategies subtle, or are they more obvious? You might also consider whether your saboteurs are of the active or passive variety. *Active saboteurs do things that aren't helpful. Passive saboteurs don't do things that would be helpful.* Try to give some serious thought to the behavior of those in your immediate network. Active saboteurs are usually a little easier to identify. A passive saboteur is simply one who could be very helpful to you if s/he did the right things, and without whose help you'd have a hard time succeeding.

Once you've tagged your saboteurs with an active or passive label, it's important to categorize them into three different groups:

- Those you can change
- Those you can avoid
- Those you can't change or avoid

You can organize your thinking by filling in the following table. Write the name of each saboteur and give some brief details about what s/he does or doesn't do that has a negative impact on your success.

Identifying your saboteurs and labeling each is important for developing your action plan, since what you do is different depending on the type of saboteur you're wrestling with. We'll take further steps to deal with saboteurs in the next chapter.

FINDING SUPPORT

Self-help books are great, but they have their limitations. Social support is a key ingredient to lifestyle change, and the ideal option would be for you to work through the Fattitudes DIET with others who can offer their help and encouragement. There are several ways you can arrange such support for yourself. First, you can look to your existing support network and determine if there's anyone who might be in the same boat as you and might want to join you in your efforts to change. A friend, perhaps? Is there someone with whom you can read this book and join efforts for mutual sharing? Or maybe your partner or spouse could be enlisted? Ideally, you would get the cooperation of those closest to you, but oftentimes they are part of the problem.

It's important to remember that the people who care about you can also be very frustrated with

MY SABOTEURS	PASSIVE SABOTEUR	ACTIVE SABOTEUR
Saboteur who can be changed		
Saboteur who can't be changed, but can be avoided		
Saboteur who can't be changed or avoided		

your self-defeating behavior. That's because they don't understand! They might very well want to help, but they don't have a clue how. The average person knows very little about the complexity of weight management, and looks at it as a simple matter of eating less and moving more. When they see you struggle, they're bewildered because they don't understand how fattitudes come into play. It's often necessary to teach your support persons how to be helpful, and many times that means helping them understand everything that's going on inside you.

If there's no one in your existing network who you can call upon, the next option is to find someone new. With a little effort, this task won't be so daunting. One option would be to look for cyber-support by visiting the Fattitudes Web site (www.fattitudes.com). Peruse the message board for individuals looking for a buddy. The Internet provides a rich source of information, and E-mail or chat-room contact that can be invaluable. Other on-line support groups can be identified at sites such as Yahoo! (dir.yahoo.com/Health) and Thrive (www.thriveonline.com).

If you have the means, and particularly if your

fattitudes seem too formidable to conquer on your own, you can consider contacting a trusted therapist. The best source of a referral would probably be your family physician or clergy, who should know about practitioners in your area as well as their specialties and reputation. When you make contact with a therapist, don't be afraid to ask questions. What is his level of experience? Has he had success with overeating clients? What is his approach? You can also ask friends for suggestions. Someone who has had a good experience with a therapist is a good source for a recommendation.

If none of these options appeals to you, don't sweat it. Thousands of people solve their own problems every day without outside help, and you could be one of them.

To help you clearly identify your primary sources of support, fill out the form on the next page.

Fattitudes
SOCIAL SUPPORT MAP

The help I need is	The person who could provide it is
_____	_____
_____	_____
_____	_____
_____	_____
_____	_____
_____	_____
_____	_____
_____	_____
_____	_____
_____	_____
_____	_____
_____	_____
_____	_____
_____	_____
_____	_____
_____	_____
_____	_____
_____	_____
_____	_____
_____	_____

THE FATTITUDES FOCUS SESSION

A crucial part of the DIET is scheduling daily time for reflection and completion of writing and other tasks. This focus session should be at least fifteen minutes long and scheduled at the beginning or end (or even better, both) of each day. This should be private time. The focus session helps you stay on track, so don't neglect it. If you find yourself lacking the time for your daily self-reflection, it's a red flag that fattitudes are afoot.

Specific tasks for the focus session may change as you work through the DIET process, but four tasks will remain constant:

- Review your day, focusing on new bits of insight, successes, and problems encountered

- Complete your daily journal

- Review your goals and strategies for developing and maintaining your fattitude-free lifestyle

- Reward yourself for positive steps taken

Always try to complete these tasks before taking on anything more specific or focused. And remember, every day! Don't let it get pushed to the wayside.

In the Discovery Phase, your focus session should also involve the following specific tasks:

- Review your daily Food-Feelings Log, trying to identify trigger situations and other emotional issues that are tied to your eating

- Review and update your list of identified fattitudes and payoffs

- Review and update your list of saboteurs and their tactics

HOW LONG WILL THIS TAKE?

It's common for clients to ask about how long they'll need to be in therapy before they "get better," and unfortunately, there usually is no good answer. There's no way to predict progress with any certainty because everyone is unique. The same is true for self-help efforts. Your rate of progress largely depends on how much effort you expend and how complicated are the issues you're confronting. Some may breeze through the four phases of the DIET and find significant benefit, while others may need to work at it longer, perhaps even starting over again and again. The best rule of thumb is, move on when you feel ready to move on, and take your progress as it comes.

To review, at the end of Discover Phase, you should have completed the following tasks:

- Sentence Completion Form
- Fattitudes Finder Form
- My Fattitudes Form
- Internal Debate Form
- My Payoffs Form
- My Saboteurs Table
- Social Support Map
- Compiled daily journal entries
- Compiled daily Food-Feelings Logs
- Daily Focus Sessions

FIVE

■

"I" IS FOR *INVENT*

By now, you should have a much better idea of the obstacles you face in trying to lose and keep weight off. You should be more aware of the connections between food and feelings, and the number of ways you use food in your efforts to cope with stress and emotions. The bulk of your old habits and food-related styles of dealing with life should be painfully apparent. At this point, many of you might be feeling that you've done nothing but make it even more obvious that healthy weight management is an impossible task—but hold on or you'll let a fattitude slip in unannounced.

Now is the time to envision a different way of doing things, to start working on new ways of coping. Don't forget, the first steps lead to the finish line.

PHASE TWO: INVENT

We often get locked into the rut of habit and ways of coping with things that aren't very effective. We continue to limp along doing the same old things because we've never considered any alternatives. That's why the fattitudes DIET challenges you to Invent new modes of thinking, feeling, and behaving.

Now that you've identified the problem areas, we challenge you to *consider the possibilities*. Now it's your time to dream. If you could be who you want to be, who would you be? How would you handle situations? What would you accomplish? What would you look like? What would be your goals, ideals, and aspirations? Close your eyes and just let yourself create an image of what you'd see in a new you.

What did you imagine? What pictures came to mind? What did you feel when you saw yourself? Let's put it on paper just to make your images more concrete.

Fattitudes
THE FATTITUDE-FREE ME FORM

I've always been

I want to be

I've always felt

I want to feel

I've always thought

I want to think

People have always
seen me as

I want people to
see me as

I've always seen
myself as

I want to see
myself as

I've never done

I want to do

It's entirely possible that you may have had difficulty imagining *anything* new because you still don't believe in your ability to change, so the Fattitude-Free Me Form would be very difficult to complete. When trying to change most of us have to deal with fear of failure and pessimism. If that's true for you, let's try to forge ahead anyhow and navigate around your old self-defeating fattitudes on the way to something new. Push yourself to dream and envision. Let yourself go, even if only for a moment.

FATTITUDE FOILERS
You've already identified your personal list of fattitudes, the old, automatic thought habits that lead you to sabotage your efforts at healthy weight management. Get out your list and look them over. Pretty potent stuff, huh? These thoughts are all too familiar to you, since you've had them clogging your brain for too many years. You probably accept them without question. It's hard for you to think of any other way to view yourself and the world. It's even harder for you to see food in a more reasonable manner. But we're going to challenge you to do just that.

Using the form below, begin creating some

Fattitudes
FATTITUDE FOILER FORM

FATTITUDE	FATTITUDE FOILER
My eating is out of control.	I make my own choices. What I eat is my own decision. I can make new choices if I learn how.

_____

_____

_____

_____

_____

_____

_____

_____

_____

_____

_____

_____

new, healthy thoughts that we'll call "fattitude foilers" because that's just what they do: They're rational thoughts that argue against the old thought habits and challenge their basis in fact. To get you started, see the example on the next page.

You might have trouble coming up with your foilers. And you certainly won't believe them when you first write them down. They'll seem weak and inadequate compared to the power of the old fattitude. That's okay. It's to be expected. Right now, your task is just to create as many foilers as you can for each fattitude. Imagine that you're in a debate class and have been asked to take the side of an issue that is new to you and contrary to what you've believed all along. Imagine how hard that would be? But also, imagine that you are able to find arguments to defend that issue. When asked to defend an opposing viewpoint you can see that view all the more clearly.

Try to make your foilers as potent as possible. Go on the attack! Fattitudes are the enemy! Beat 'em to hell and back! Use whatever argument ammunition you can muster to counter them. Find examples to bolster your contrary position. You can do it! The more substantial and plentiful your foilers, the stronger they'll be when we put them to work in Phase Three.

NEEDS AND NUTRITION

By using your Food-Feelings Logs you've become more aware of the reasons *why* you eat. You've been able to identify some trigger situations, and some feelings and needs that lead you to overeat. Eating has become an automatic way of dealing with your emotional life but it's not the most healthy alternative. Next, let's clarify the needs that underlie your eating, and consider better ways to meet those needs.

Here's a work sheet that will help in this process.

As with your foiler list, the more alternative coping techniques you can generate, the better. The bottom line is that if you can decrease your reliance on food to meet your emotional needs, you'll be more successful at weight management. Another way to put this is that if you recognize your needs and feelings, you'll be able to make a choice about how to cope, and choose some method other than overeating.

Dawn identified that she usually overate when she came home from a busy, frantic day at her clerical job and ran smack into her two teenage sons expecting to be fed before their evening extracurricular activities. Being a guilt-ridden single parent,

COPING ALTERNATIVES FORM

I usually eat when I need/feel/want:	What I can do instead of eating is:
_____	_____
_____	_____
_____	_____
_____	_____
_____	_____
_____	_____
_____	_____
_____	_____
_____	_____
_____	_____
_____	_____
_____	_____
_____	_____
_____	_____
_____	_____
_____	_____

Dawn felt it was her responsibility to give the boys what they needed, so she would usually drop everything and march into the kitchen to begin cooking dinner. While cooking, she nibbled, stuffed, and generally crammed whatever was available into her mouth without realizing what she was doing.

As she began to tune into the feelings surrounding her binges, Dawn became aware that she was feeling frustrated and overwhelmed by the demands of running a household by herself. What she really needed was help. After we discussed how she might meet her needs more directly, she began to require her sons' assistance in the kitchen with all the meal preparations. Although the teens grudgingly cooperated, the pre-meal teamwork soon turned into a pleasant time for sharing as well as making the chores of cooking, serving, and cleaning a much more efficient process.

It's important to remember, though, that most overeaters give up their dependence on food only when they feel ready to do so. And they can only feel ready when they have something else to turn to. Emotional overeating won't go away until you replace it with more effective coping techniques. The process of change can lead to a very unsettling period of time during which food begins to lose its emotional power, but you have yet to trust your new coping skills. This is a transition period, one that usually precedes a turning point for the better. If you find yourself in this bind, don't worry; it means you're on the right track.

FIGHTING FAT WITH FATS

As we stated previously, there are many similarities among emotional overeaters. In fact, there are four specific coping skills we call FATS that are crucial to a healthy relationship with food, but are commonly lacking among those who eat for emotional reasons. These four skills are:

- Feelings expression
- Assertiveness
- Time management
- Self-care

Overeaters usually hide their feelings from others and usually don't set effective limits. They're so low on the priority list that they usually run out of time to meet their own needs. And they usually take care of everybody but themselves. This four-pronged pattern usually results in much bottled-up anger and resentment, along with overreliance on food to keep feelings out. Mastering FATS is a key step toward ending an unhealthy relationship with food. These four skills are so important that we'll spend time explaining how to deal with each one in detail.

FEELINGS EXPRESSION:
BOTTLING UP IS BAD FOR YOU

Emotional overeaters don't have an easy time handling their emotional lives. They tend to be frightened of letting feelings go and have few emotional outlets. Since feelings are often so unknown and scary, overeaters tend to use food as a generic emotional stuffer so feelings don't sneak out by mistake, which leads to both stress and weight gain.

Being overweight carries enough health risks on its own, but there is also research that points out that bottling up feelings is bad for your body. This is particularly true for bottled-up anger, which has been shown to have a hand in causing heart problems such as high blood pressure and arterial blockage. Women are especially at risk for the harmful physical effects of squashed anger. Having emotional upsets is not the problem, it's what we do with the feelings.

What obstacles keep you from being more open with your feelings? Are you afraid of what will happen if you "let go"? Do you worry whether your feelings are legitimate, or "right"? Do you fear being rejected or abandoned if you show your true feelings to others? Do you fear being judged as weak or inadequate if your tears break through? If you think about these obstacles, you may be able to identify some new fattitudes like "If I let my feelings out, people will be disgusted with me and will turn away."

There are many modes of emotional expression. The most common, and the one most problematic for most of us, is talking things out. Saying what we feel to another person is a risk many folks find too difficult to take. We all know how hard it can be to say, "I love you," or even worse, "I need you." These are risky phrases in a world that all too often can be hurtful and rejecting. So many of us confuse "strength" with "stoicism" because it seems that we're less likely to be hurt if we just lie low and follow the safe, silent path.

Let's write again. Use the following form to identify our goal and the obstacles to expressing your feelings.

Fattitudes

FEELINGS EXPRESSION EXPLORATION
FORM

I have most
trouble expressing

Some ways I could
express this are

What I'd like
to say most is

What makes this
so difficult is

The person I have the most
trouble with is

What makes this person
so difficult is

The biggest fear
I have is

Ways I can overcome
this fear are

Another helpful exercise is to generate a list of expressive activities. In addition to talking, what are some other ways you can get your feelings out? What things do you like to do that help you "unload"? How do you get relief? An expressive activity could be anything, like playing a game, doing a craft, exercising, etc. For some folks, it might be necessary to invent a new activity, one that you've not tried before. What works for you?

Later on, we'll take discuss some letter-writing tasks that will aid your feelings expression skills.

ASSERTIVENESS: I HAVE NEEDS, TOO

Another major skill that overeaters tend to find lacking or weak in their repertoire is asserting their needs. Assertiveness is a key ingredient to dealing with just about any situation that involves another person, whether it be at home, on the job, or in an intimate relationship.

There's a lot of confusion about assertiveness, however. Being assertive is very often mistaken as being aggressive, and vice versa. Assertiveness is not the same as aggressiveness. Being assertive means that you're able to speak up and take action to defend your own rights without infringing on the rights or dignity of others. The aggressive person may get his way, but he steps on others to accomplish that goal. He takes care of his own needs at the expense of those around him. The aggressive person makes waves that others find hard to navigate. Aggressiveness leads to hurt, anger, and resentment.

At the other end of the spectrum is the passive individual who usually says and does nothing to stand up for herself, gets taken advantage of, then feels secretly resentful and ashamed. Passive people end up feeling like doormats for everyone else, and feel self-critical because they can't avoid the "victim" role. Passive people usually wear a smile on their faces and a secret frown in their hearts.

Many of us vacillate between the extremes of passivity and aggressiveness, staying quiet and holding things in until a small event triggers a volcanic eruption. This scenario leads to everyone feeling badly in the end. Even doormats get worn out after a period of time, and explosions of anger over past mistreatment can be quite impressive.

Assertiveness, on the other hand, isn't loud. It doesn't hurt. It doesn't require great strength or presidential debate techniques. It doesn't mean you'll lose friends and create enemies. Assertiveness means you can ask for what you want and say no to what you don't want. It means you can set a limit so that your needs don't get trampled on, but it also means you can be helpful if you choose to do so. Assertiveness means you can express your needs and wants in a way that results in satisfaction to everyone concerned. It doesn't mean you become a selfish, exploitative person.

Behaving assertively is a foreign concept to almost all emotional eaters. You can probably stop right now and think of a hundred situations in which you'd like to behave assertively, but for whatever reason have not. Can you think of times when you've felt your needs ignored? When you've done something you really didn't want to do and felt angry at yourself for doing it, and angry at the person you did it for? Can you think of people with whom you have the most trouble speaking up for yourself? What are they like? What do they do to cause you to withdraw or back down?

Becoming appropriately assertive takes a lot of work. You first must convince yourself that your needs and feelings are legitimate and worth taking a stand for. Then, you have to find the right words and the right body language to maximize the effectiveness of your communication. Next, it's a matter of taking the risk and trying a new approach to dealing with troublesome situations. It's a scary step.

Most people fumble around for a while as they attempt new behavior. Often, there's the tendency to overcorrect: A person who has behaved passively most of her life might jump too far into aggressiveness. If this happens, no sweat. As they say, practice makes perfect.

We'll work more in the next chapter on actions you can take to build assertiveness. Right now, just work on getting your thoughts in order about how you've been in the past and how you want to be in the future. You can use the Assertive Situations Form to help in this effort. Think of the typical situations where you behave too passively or too aggressively. Who are the people with whom you have the most difficulty? Write it all down.

TIME MANAGEMENT:
LIVING IN A 24-HOUR DAY

Another major skill deficit for most emotional eaters has to do with how they manage their limited time. We all try to juggle too much at one time and usually end up feeling like most of what we need to do goes undone. This is particularly true if

Assertive Situations Form

I don't act assertively when   **What I'd like to say/do is**

_____

_____

_____

_____

_____

_____

_____

_____

_____

_____

_____

_____

_____

_____

you're working, trying to raise a family, and trying to maintain a household. There never seems to be enough time to get everything accomplished, and typically we go to bed thinking about how behind we are. Remember the catchy paperweight saying? "The harder I work, the behinder I get."

Emotional eaters tend to expect too much of themselves. As we discussed earlier, most overeaters have low self-esteem, and one way they try to compensate for this feeling of inadequacy is to be overly pleasing to others. They try to make up for their perceived deficiencies by currying the favor of everyone. Because they want to make a good impression, or because they're afraid of being seen as the unworthy person they feel themselves to be, overeaters take on the burdens of others and have a hard time saying "no" to requests. As a result, their schedules become more and more cluttered with tasks that all vie for positions of high priority, which then leads to frustration, stress, and, ironically, even lower self-esteem. There's never enough time to be everything to everybody.

The key to effective time management is to decide what's *really* important and what's not. Establish a pecking order of priorities and allocate your limited time so that you focus your efforts on the most essential tasks. When handling many complex demands, it's necessary to have a written schedule, with time divided according to a task's position on the priority list. A common experience for one who has too many "highest priority" tasks is to consider any new challenge insurmountable, which then leads to immobilization and, of course, not getting anything done.

I had one client who was working on time management skills. I asked her to bring to session a list of things she expected herself to accomplish on the coming Saturday, which was the day she reserved for errands and household chores she was unable to accomplish during her hectic work week. When she showed me the list, it was two pages long! I immediately suggested she should hire a team of contractors, since that was the only way she would check off everything on the list. With some work, we were able to divide the long list into groups of "A" and "B" and "C" priorities, which then made things a lot more manageable. My client was able to see how she had always managed her time in an unrealistic and haphazard manner, which typically led her to feeling frustrated, discouraged, and beset with an overwhelming urge to binge. When she tackled only the "A" priority tasks, she was able to get them

Fattitudes
DAILY TASK LIST

Things I must get done today ("A" priority) are

Things I'd like to get done but might not have the time for ("B" priority) are

Things I'd like to get done but that could definitely wait ("C" priority) are

all done (and even got to a few of the "B" list). Despite not being able to check off everything, she had a successful day—successful enough that her urge to overeat did not appear.

Give some serious thought to your time and how you manage it. Are your expectations realistic? Do you expect too much from yourself? How many "A" priority items crowd the top of your list? Try writing down your daily schedule and make a task list to get an idea of where you get overloaded and where you waste time that could be spent more productively somewhere else. Try the following form and see if it helps in your planning.

We'll take action on your time management plan in the next chapter.

SELF-CARE: THE ANTIDOTE TO EXHAUSTION

If you're beginning to see some overlap among the FATS skills, you're right on the mark. Weakness in the four FATS skills makes up what can be considered the prototypical personality style of the emotional over-eater: a self-sacrificing, bottled-up, overwhelmed individual who puts everybody else's needs first and ends up frustrated, guilt-ridden, and hungry.

The biggest skill deficit—the one with the most destructive impact—is the emotional eater's self-neglect. Emotional eaters tend to treat themselves and their bodies with contempt; they view their own needs as unimportant and spend no time in activities that would be restorative and self-nurturing. I've worked in a number of inpatient mental health units, and although there's a diverse range of diagnoses among those that require hospitalization, the common thread among them all is a lack of self-care. If you don't take care of your own needs, no one will do it for you, and you'll end up broken-down and depleted.

At the root of the emotional eater's self-neglect is an inner feeling of unworthiness and self-hatred. It's very common for an emotional eater to neglect basic self-care and health-related tasks. I can recall one Fattitudes group, comprised of seven women. At one session the topic of self-neglect came up. During the discussion I asked how many of them had done a recent self-breast exam. Each woman admitted that she'd *never* done one. When we discussed the reasons underlying the omission of this basic health care behavior, we uncovered the depths of the bodily disgust that had led all of them to avoid touching themselves. One woman confessed that "I don't exist from the neck down." She said she could look in a mirror and not see the lower ninety-five percent of her body, so it wasn't surprising to her that she'd never thought to examine her breasts as a preventive measure.

At the end of this poignant group session, I quickly made a breast self-exam a homework assignment for everyone, and the next session we discussed everyone's experiences. A few were unable to complete the task the first time, but everyone was eventually successful. It was a first step toward treating themselves with enough respect to make healthy decisions about how to live.

To ensure effective self-care you must disconnect it from the idea of being "selfish." Self-care and selfishness are two very different concepts. The selfish individual exploits others for her personal gain, while one who is good at self-care balances the needs of others with her own needs for self-nurturing. There are many individuals who are hardworking folks who go the extra mile for others, but they are also committed to taking care of their own needs so they have something left to give.

Self-care is often something emotional eaters must approach one step at a time, because as a new habit it feels rather odd. Now ask yourself what needs do you routinely neglect? In what ways do you allow other people's needs and wants to override your own? What activities do you see others engaging in that are enjoyable and soothing, yet you never allow yourself to do the same? What things could you do to honor your body instead of beating it up as you typically do? It may seem to you that self-care is too far down the road to ever achieve. But, take a first step. Generate a list of self-soothing and self-nurturing activities.

The first time through this form you'll probably end up with many more entries on the left side than on the right. Yes, this is a difficult task. You'll probably have to stretch yourself. Maybe it would help to think of a friend who seems to take good care of herself. What does she do? How does she spend her time? Think of things you've always wanted to do but never "got around to." After you've thought hard on this matter, go back to your list and make sure you've got *twice* the number of nurturing activities to neglectful ones. Don't stop until you've really pushed your limits in coming up with them. Then set the list aside; we'll use it later.

Mastering the FATS coping skills will help you take a major step toward ending your cycle of self-defeat with weight management. Now is the time to start thinking about and practicing your new skills. In the next chapter we'll help you put them into action.

"I" Is for *Invent*

SELF-CARE ACTIVITIES LIST

I neglect myself in these ways:	I could do these things to self-nurture:

TACKLING THE PAYOFFS OF POUNDS

By now you should have some ideas about hidden payoffs motivating you to avoid weight loss. Payoffs can range in "size" from those that are small and easily surmountable to those that are enormous and seemingly impossible to dismantle. For example, the payoff "If I stay fat, I won't have to buy new clothes" might seem insignificant compared to "If I stay fat, my husband will remain distant and I won't have to feel anxious about sexual matters." The existence of significant payoffs can be the most formidable of all obstacles to healthy weight management. Whenever I work with a client on weight issues who continues to show no progress, it's almost always because there's a hidden payoff or two that has not yet been identified.

More often than not, discovering hidden payoffs means revisiting the traumatic events or relationships that first brought about the need for weight gain, which is often quite painful. Resolving payoffs requires that we reckon with the past and/or the present so that the payoff can be removed as a motivating force.

Maria became aware that she used her weight as an excuse for feeling depressed and for remaining detached from others. As long as she was overweight, she had a good reason to feel badly and to explain her social isolation, and also didn't need to look further into her problems. She had been traumatized by her ex-husband's extramarital affair that led to their painful divorce. Focusing on her weight problems protected her from recognizing that she had been depressed about this for many years. As she began to address her unresolved feelings of loss, rejection, and anger, she was able to convince herself that she had the strength to face the past and move on to the possibility of a new relationship. As she neutralized the power of the payoff, she was gradually able to adopt a healthier lifestyle, and eventually to lose weight.

Does eliminating payoffs require psychotherapy? Not necessarily, although the answer depends on the complexity of the obstacle and whether one can address it fully without assistance. Recent research has shown that writing can be useful in improving emotional and even physical health, by helping individuals confront unresolved feelings.

Do you have feelings from the past that you've never addressed? Do your payoffs relate to events that you've not faced? Are there old traumas still lurking within you? If so, we'll need to get you to put some things on paper. Try writing a letter to your fat entitled "I hate you, don't leave me." Say whatever you choose. We'll do some more writing aimed at helping heal past hurts in the chapter that follows.

STIFLING THE SABOTEURS

In Phase One you gave some thought to those around you who have a destructive impact on your weight management attempts. We asked you to tag your saboteurs as active or passive and then to categorize them into three categories: those you can change, those you can avoid, and those you can't change or avoid.

Now, it's time to give some thought to a plan to deal effectively with these saboteurs. This plan will require building upon your FATS coping skills. Stifling a saboteur will depend upon your ability to assertively communicate and express feelings, and to set limits with those in your support network. The ultimate goal of working with saboteurs is to end their negative influence on your weight management efforts and, if possible, turn them into supporters.

Take another look at the Saboteurs Table you completed in Chapter Four. The best type of saboteur to have in your midst, clearly, is one who can be changed. Changeable saboteurs are those who are willing to listen to your feedback and can be

"I" Is for *Invent*
Letter To My Fat

Dear Fat: I hate you, don't leave me. _____

_____

_____

_____

_____

_____

_____

_____

_____

_____

_____

_____

_____

_____

_____

_____

_____

_____

_____

_____

motivated to do things differently. Saboteurs may not always be aware that what they do is harmful to your efforts, so communicating with the saboteur and clearly relating your wants and needs is an important step.

What do they do that's harmful to your success? What don't they do that would be helpful? What specific things could they do that would keep you on track? It's important to be specific. Organize your thoughts and feelings with the following form.

If a saboteur can't be changed or is unwilling to change, but can be avoided without causing you further problems, restructure your social contacts so that the saboteur is a less prominent figure in your daily life. Spend less time with these people, find a way to disconnect from those who hurt you the most. This is often difficult, because saboteurs generally have some emotional connection to you and won't just fade into the woodwork willingly. Your growing skills in setting limits will get frequent challenges!

The most potentially destructive of all saboteurs are those you can't change and can't avoid. These are the folks who are more or less fixed parts of your social life and who can't be convinced to behave toward you in a more helpful manner. There is no clear-cut solution in this situation, but efforts can be made

SUPPORT SOLICITATION FORM

Your help is important to me because

The things that you do that aren't helpful are

What I really need and want from you is

What I'm willing to do for you in return is

to insulate yourself from the impact. Revise your hopes and expectations of them. Waiting for something that's not going to happen—their behavior changing—is a waste of time. Also, step up efforts to locate supporters who can buffer the impact of a saboteur.

THE FATTITUDES FOCUS SESSION, PHASE TWO

As in the discovery phase, you should be scheduling daily fifteen-minute times during which you do nothing but think about yourself and your progress in fighting your fattitudes. A red fattitudes flag should pop up when you find other activities shoving your focus session out of the way. This time is crucial to your continuing progress. See page 125 to review your standard tasks.

To foster your development of FATS coping skills during this phase, you might try using the following to spur your journal entries.

In addition, during your focus sessions you should

- Continue to review daily food-feelings logs to find connections between eating and emotional triggers

- Review progress in finding nonfood ways to meet your unmet needs.

To review, at the end of the Invent phase you should have completed the following tasks:

- The Fattitude-Free Me Form
- Fattitude Foiler Form
- Coping Alternatives Form
- Feelings Expression Exploration Form
- Assertive Situations Form
- Daily Task List
- Self-Care Activities List
- Dear Fat letter
- Support Solicitation Form
- Daily Focus sessions

Fattitudes

JOURNAL ENTRY

I need to express my feelings about

I need to be more assertive by

I need to manage my time better by

I need to nurture myself by

SIX

■

"E" IS FOR *EXTINGUISH*

Do you feel as if you're getting somewhere? You may still have doubts, which is perfectly reasonable. You're tackling a formidable foe: years and years of habit and failure that won't die easily. Modifying your lifestyle is very difficult, and it doesn't occur overnight. So be realistic and avoid expectations that are akin to diet mentality fattitudes: remember change requires chipping away, not chainsawing.

Take a moment and review what you've accomplished so far. You've gotten to know yourself a little better and have illuminated the connections between food and feelings. You've done a good job finding a big chunk of your fattitudes, and have identified some hidden payoffs for remaining overweight. You've also learned about weaknesses you probably have in crucial FATS coping skills, and you've located weight management saboteurs in your social network.

In addition, you've begun to develop a plan for healthy thinking that will help fight and foil your fattitudes. You've identified some alternate ways of meeting your needs that don't rely on eating, and you've created a plan for getting the support you need to be successful. Sounds like you've done some work, doesn't it? Let's do some more.

PHASE THREE: *EXTINGUISH*

Now we get into the meat of changing. Or maybe we should say into the *fat* of changing, since the fat is what we want to go away. One of my clients was feeling frustrated with how hard it was to end self-defeating behavior and said, "I wish there was a way you could just suck all this crap out of my brain so I'd be different by tomorrow morning." I thought for a moment, then asked, "Sort of like liposuction, huh?" The client nodded, then said, "Yeah. But we'd have to call it *psycho*suction."

Psychosuction doesn't exist in our current state of medical technology, and it would likely be very messy anyhow. So, we're stuck with the less miraculous methods that require elbow grease and persistence. What we do in Phase Three is work at **Extinguishing** your old patterns of thinking, feeling, and behaving while we attempt to replace them with the new, healthy patterns that you invented in Phase Two. Remember, chip, don't chainsaw. Let's plow forward.

FOIL 'EM, THEN FORGET 'EM

One of the best places to start with lifestyle change is inside your head. Life is ninety-five percent attitude, and weight loss is almost all fattitude. Changing the way you think and interpret situations, or altering your "self-talk," is a crucial first step toward behaving in successful ways. Human beings have a powerful tool in their ability to consciously rethink and reinterpret events. Just consider how easy it is to worry yourself into a tizzy, even when there's no objective reason to be concerned. If you take on a crisis mentality, you can think yourself into a panic attack.

If you stop and deliberately try to take a different perspective (by substituting alternate thoughts and self-talk phrases), you can have a substantial impact on your emotions and behaviors. This isn't easy by any means, because you're trying to tackle thought patterns that are automatic and reflexive. But all that means is that you have to try extra hard if you're to win the war.

To foil and forget your fattitudes, you're going to have to engage in daily self-monitoring, which means that you have to watch yourself as if you're a private detective on a surveillance mission. Whenever you catch yourself engaging in a fattitude frenzy, quickly move to substitute these thoughts with the foilers you invented earlier. Fight back! If necessary, carry your list of fattitude foilers around with you, so that you have some alternate perspectives to employ in your own best interest. You can beat those bullies. Don't let them push you around!

People who can look on the "bright side," those optimistic folks who always seem to have a smile on their faces, are better off in many ways than the rest of us. They're usually happier and healthier in the long run. Positive thinking is a virtue and an excellent way of dealing with life. But fighting your fattitudes requires taking a more specific and targeted approach than just thinking positively, since fattitudes are generally complex and deeply rooted patterns that defy simple solutions.

Your plan to foil 'em and forget 'em should include continuing to keep track of emotional triggers for overeating. It's also important to record your "fattitude fits" and write down the fattitude foilers you employed to fight back. Try using a format such as the one on the next page.

This may seem a bit tedious, but in the beginning it's important to make your efforts at change as concrete as you can, to increase their power. Perhaps later, as you get the hang of it, keeping such a detailed log will become unnecessary, as you'll be closer to making fattitude foiling more habitual and automatic. But for now, write everything down.

DEALING WITH THE DEMONS

When you found your hidden payoffs, you probably found your demons as well. As repeated throughout this book, your problems with overeating probably have roots in past events and relationships, many from as far back as childhood. Can things that happened so long ago still be affecting us? The answer is a resounding yes. I've had a number of clients in

Fattitudes
FOIL 'EM AND FORGET 'EM FORM

DATE_____

Time	Fattitude Detected	Foiler Employed

their forties and fifties who lamented the fact that they still worried about pleasing their parents. We're all products of our pasts, and when we don't deal with things effectively when they occur, they surface later to bother us again. Such is the human psyche.

How do we deal with the demons? How do we put to rest the troubles that still haunt us? Sometimes it may require psychotherapy. But often there are ways to heal on our own. And one of the best ways, again, is writing.

A technique I've used with many clients is to help them identify the people with whom they have unfinished business. Then they must take steps to express what had never before been expressed, put the past behind, and get on track with healthy living. One of the best ways to accomplish this is by writing unsent letters.

An unsent letter is just what it sounds like: a letter written to a specific person that you may or may not intend to send, depending on what would be most helpful to you. The act of writing to a specific person brings us face-to-face with feelings we may have avoided for many years. It's often a painful process that we put off because we don't want to feel the pain. One client tried and failed for several weeks to pick up pen and paper to write a letter to her parents, who had been alcoholic and neglectful and who still refused to take any responsibility for their behavior during the client's formative years. After she was able to get something written, it took another several weeks before she felt ready to read it aloud in session. When she did, it brought a flood of tears. She had a hard time getting through the entire letter and had to spread it over several appointments. She found that the experience was relieving. When she was finished, though, she clearly felt as if she'd gotten something burdensome off her chest. Soon thereafter, she reported noticing that her urge to overeat when thinking of or having contact with her parents decreased. Writing and reading the letter wasn't a miracle cure, because she had much more work to do, but it was a solid step toward healing. Here's what she wrote:

To Mom and Dad,
It's hard for me to even start this letter, because to call you "mom" and "dad" seems so unde- served. All my life I've spent waiting for the love that never comes. All my life I've spent trying one thing after another, trying to figure out what it takes to be loved by you. I've never gotten there.

Do you realize how much I hurt? Do you know what it was like to lie in bed and cry myself to sleep? Do you know how much I ached to be held and comforted, but all you did was criticize and walk away? I grew up hating myself for being so useless, when I should have been hating you all along.

I see now that you both had problems. I see now why Dad touched me only to hit me and punish me. I see now why Mom had to hide in her gin bottle because she felt so alone and unloved, too. I try to forgive you for the lies and the hurt, but still I hope someday you'll be different. I know now that I eat to give myself what I can't get from you, what I could never get from you. I hate you for what you did to me. You've left me with a hole in my heart that I fear I will never fill. I feel alone in this battle to save my own life. The damage feels so great. If only we could have been friends, things would have been so different.

I hope to learn how to be a friend to myself. I hope to learn how to let others in so I can feel their compassion. I will be different someday. I wonder if you'll notice?

Another technique is to write to yourself or a troublesome aspect of yourself. One common approach is to write to the feelings within that affect your self-esteem. Although it's almost a cliché in our society to speak of the "inner child," a majority of my clients refer to a feeling that there is a part of themselves that never had the right nurturing to grow up into a healthy adult. They feel a big part of themselves got left behind somewhere along the way. When someone writes to her inner self it is often an illuminating and helpful process.

Glenna considered herself a "hopeless case." She suffered from a severely negative self-image that led her to act with self-hatred so regularly that taking care of herself was a foreign concept to her. Her journey to health was arduous and slow, but she was able to foster her growth by writing to the lonely, neglected little girl she felt could never measure up to her parents' expectations. Her initial effort in this process was as follows:

To my Inner Self:
I always thought of you as my monster lurking within. It is for that very reason that I beat you, fought you, hated you, and tried to get rid of you. For that I would like to deeply apologize.

All of my life, you were my inner voice trying to sabotage any little happiness I could find. Whenever I looked for someone to console me or understand me and couldn't find anyone, I would try to take it out on you. I thought it was your fault. I know now that you, too, need to be consoled and understood. You were lonely and desperate for something to grasp on to. Neither of us had parents who were available to us psychologically or physically. We were both very angry and have spent a lifetime in fear and frustration.

The one difference that you have, that I will never have with my parents, is that I want to be your friend. I want to understand you and nurture you. I want to make up for the time lost together. I will never be able to do that with my parents, but I always want to know that you and I will be here for each other. I never realized that all those times I feared and hated you, you were only feelings I had internalized within myself. If I would have stopped being so angry with you I might have realized that you only wanted to help me. You were just as lonely as I was. If only I could have noticed. I was too busy being wrapped up in self-pity to realize that you needed me every bit as much as I needed you.

The constant fear and loneliness that we both feel is not your fault. I know that we could have helped each other. We still need to help each other. We need to work together to become one.

I spent a lifetime abusing you with food to keep you quiet. It didn't work because it was really me you needed instead. I abused you in the same way I was taught. I didn't know any better.

I'm sorry, so truly sorry for not being the parent you needed just like I needed. We have so much to fight yet, but I hope we can do it together.

One of my clients, during her struggle to resolve past hurts that continued to plague her life, asked, "Why can't my emotional pain go away like my physical pain does? When I broke my leg, I put it in a cast, stayed off of it, and in about six weeks it healed itself. Why don't my emotional wounds do the same damned thing?" I sympathized with her and wished, too, that things were so designed. But, of course, they're not.

Write as many letters as you need to begin to feel some resolution. Set them down for a day. Reread them. Then, write some more. Face things head-on. You can do it.

FATS TO THE RESCUE

Now is the time to put into action your game plan to master Feelings expression, Assertiveness, Time management, and Self-care. Like any skill, these require practice, practice, practice, and you can expect your first efforts to be not as polished as your later ones. You'll be hesitant. You'll be scared. You'll make mistakes. But don't back away from the challenge.

ACTIVITIES FOR EXPRESSING YOUR FEELINGS

Previously, you identified the feelings that you have difficulty expressing on a day-to-day basis. You identified the reasons why you tend to keep these feelings to yourself. You also gave some thought to ways that you feel comfortable getting your feelings out. What are they? Is it talking with a friend? Taking a walk? Gardening? Playing a sport? What haven't you done, but need to do? Who is it you most need to communicate with?

Take another look at the list of feelings expression activities you created earlier. It's time to get moving. It's time to take action for change. Where do you want to begin? What's your first step? Each day you must set the goal of engaging in at least one expressive activity. Whatever you decide to do, make sure it's an activity that lightens your emotional load and relieves you of something normally held inside.

Your expressive activity may overlap with other FATS skills, such as your choosing to talk with a friend about something that has been bothering you about the relationship. That's fine. All the FATS skills interact and combine in how you live your daily life. Just as weakness in one area can produce weakness in another, strengthening in one can lead to growth in another.

Della's story highlights the importance of expressing your feelings daily. Della was a married woman with three grown children. She had been a full time mother since graduating from college with a degree in art, and came to counseling because of chronic emotional eating, depression, and bottled-up anger. As we talked, it became clear that her artwork, which had always been a way she found her own "special place," was something she was actively avoiding. Whenever she attempted to draw or paint she would get a feeling of being physically "weighted down"—to the point that lifting a brush or pencil was impossible. With some work, she discovered that one of the major blocks to her artwork was her fear of the feelings she might express on the canvas.

One day, she was feeling particularly frustrated and decided to force herself to paint. What began as a cheerful, lighthearted abstract combining yellow, green, and other pastels slowly took the shape of a reddened face with black outlines and an open mouth that appeared to be screaming. When Della was finished, she was struck by the intensity of the picture and then realized that she had painted her own anger, anger at all those who pushed their needs onto her and expected that she respond like a dutiful servant. A primary target of her anger was her husband, whom she saw as both dependent and self-centered, and whom she also saw as unwilling to change. Although she recognized that improving her marriage was not totally within her control, she vowed that her artwork was her "salvation" and that she would no longer deny herself such a crucial expressive activity. Once she had taken this step, her overeating gradually faded away.

Remember, perform at least one expressive activity per day. Have fun!

ASSERTIVENESS ACTIVITIES

Just like most behavior changes, becoming more assertive begins with practice, risk-taking, and trial and error. Take another look at the Assertive Situations Form you completed in Chapter Five. In filling it out you've already given thought to problem situations in which you need to do a better job of setting limits, communicating your needs, and addressing things more directly with others. It's a truism that the more you open your mouth to speak, the less you'll open it to overeat.

What's your plan of action? Have you ranked your situations in order of their difficulty? What situation should be your first step toward assertive communication? It's best to start with one that's lower on the complexity list and build your confidence step by step. Many people feel it's easier to begin skill-building by first addressing situations that don't involve a personal relationship.

For example, suppose you're out for dinner at a nice restaurant and your meal has been uneven in quality. What do most of us say when the waiter asks us, "How is everything?" We usually smile and say everything's just great (i.e., we take the passive road out), but we leave vowing never to return. We could also choose to ventilate our frustration in a hostile manner (i.e., an aggressive mode) by saying something like "The food stinks and so do you." Why not just tell the truth, but do so in a diplomatic and courteous manner? Why not take a simple action that might salvage the dining experience while giving the restaurant valuable customer feedback?

When the waiter asks for your feedback, say, "Thank you for asking. I've been to this restaurant several times in the past and have had a great meal every time. Tonight, though, I've not been as pleased. The baked potato and salad were excellent, but the steak was overdone and grisly." In this situation, everybody wins. Your waiter will benefit, as will the restaurant, and you'll benefit by learning to voice your feelings more effectively—and maybe getting the offending steak taken off your bill. This little vignette illustrates a common and effective technique for giving constructive criticism called "stroke and poke," which means that you provide positive feedback first (i.e., stroke), then give the negative (i.e., poke), which helps balance your message and makes it easier to hear. Begin by looking for situations like the above to practice your new skills.

Behaving assertively in personal situations is more challenging because the stakes are higher. We get concerned about hurting feelings, getting rejected, or ruining relationships. We fear that the retribution for our action will be more severe than the benefit of taking it. We let things build up until everything comes out in a big explosion, which leaves everybody feeling badly. The anxiety that surrounds being assertive with a friend or loved one is often quite uncomfortable. It leads to awkwardness when we try to express ourselves, and often causes us to say things a bit more harshly than we should. Again, practice is the key to becoming effectively assertive.

Have you identified a personal situation in which you need to behave assertively? One that requires you to end your old patterns of relating and try something new? Is it scary to think about? Why? What are the thoughts that occur to you as you consider what to do? What fears do you have? On a more positive note, what benefits will accrue to both you and the other person if you speak up? How does everyone win?

Belinda had a very tough situation to deal with, one that she had avoided and lived with (although not happily) for many years. She worked part-time and was a mother with two young children. Her husband worked full-time and felt that his duties ended when he got home. After eight years of marriage, Belinda felt overwhelmed with the responsibilities of her job as well as bearing the full brunt of child-rearing and household tasks. She also had no time for taking care of herself. Not surprisingly, Belinda binged because it was the only pleasure she afforded herself and because it helped her stuff down her resentment at her husband, who sat watching TV and drinking beer most of the evening while she scurried around the house trying to keep up.

Belinda was angry at the uneven division of labor, but she was also fearful of taking assertive steps because her husband had a bad temper, especially after that third beer. She'd already had a few angry explosions about his lack of involvement but her husband hadn't been motivated to change. She realized she needed to communicate her needs more effectively or her marriage would continue to disintegrate because of her anger and dissatisfaction.

One day she felt courageous enough to take a first step. When her husband arrived home, before he'd grabbed the first beer from the fridge, she put her arms around him and said, "Honey, I really need your help. Can you help David with his homework while I cook dinner?" Her husband was irritated at first, but he did do as asked. Later that same evening, Belinda asked him to supervise the children's baths. Her husband protested at first, with irritation, but she asked him again the same way, and he eventually got up to help. This was the beginning of Belinda's learning to speak up for her own needs without being afraid of getting hurt. As she experienced more and more success with assertiveness, her confidence grew and her need to overeat dropped off.

The key to becoming more assertive is to plan your steps, practice in advance, and expect to make mistakes until you really get the hang of it. Your self-esteem, your relationships, and your waistline will all benefit from your new skills in communicating. Try tackling at least one assertiveness challenge each day until you get the hang of it.

TIME MANAGEMENT ACTIVITIES

It's time to get out paper and pencil once again and get a detailed look at how you spend your waking hours. Let's take a day-by-day approach and sort through all the demands on your schedule to see if there are ways to achieve the goals of getting what you need done, meeting the needs of others, and saving time to rest, relax, and recreate.

As you did in Phase Two by completing the Daily Task List, begin by making a list of tasks and goals that you would like to accomplish tomorrow. Generate the list in no particular order, just off the top of your head. Once you're finished, stop and take a look at it. It's probably lengthy. Reduce the list's complexity by categorizing each task as an "A" or "B" or "C" priority by ranking and comparing. Ask yourself, what can wait? What can be put off without causing additional stress? What *really* needs your immediate attention? Revise your prioritization accordingly, and make sure at least one self-care task is assigned to the "A" group (even if you have to fudge a little).

Next, map out a schedule for your day. Assign time to each task depending upon its priority and complexity. What time do you have to get started? Where do you have to be at what time of day? Have you built in enough flex time to handle surprises? Have you created a day that's unrealistic to complete? Where's your down time? What tasks will just have to wait until another day?

William was a high-powered executive who had both a weight problem and a time problem. His days were long and frenetic, and he usually left work around seven or eight in the evening feeling drained and tense. He was on blood pressure medication and feared having a heart attack, especially since cardiac disease ran in his family. On his way home he typically stopped by a fast-food drive-thru and binged on cheeseburgers, his first meal of the day since early morning coffee and donuts. When we looked closely at his daily schedule, it was clear that his perfectionism and need for complete control resulted in his inability to delegate tasks. He was a micro-manager, and he felt regularly overwhelmed by obligations that could not be neglected. Although his overeating was connected to other problems as well, his time management was also a significant component. He worked intensively to improve the situation and later was able to approach his work responsibilities in a more realistic and effective manner.

Each day, create a Daily Task List and schedule for yourself until you're able to plan things in your mind and still maintain an organized approach to getting things done. Remember: Make time for what's really important.

SELF-CARE ACTIVITIES

You've already done some heavy-duty thinking about ways you tend to neglect your own needs. You've also tried to generate a list of things you could do to nurture yourself and meet your own needs. Are you ready to give it a try? Are you ready to take steps to break the old self-hatred cycle of self-abuse and treat yourself like a deserving human being? Have you convinced yourself that you need good things just as much as your next-door neighbor does?

Sometimes, when you're dealing with automatic behaviors like self-neglect, forging ahead, even when you don't feel completely convinced of your inner worth, is the ticket to success. Taking a risk and trying on something new can help create a break in an otherwise self-perpetuating cycle. And that break, even if it's minuscule to begin with, is what we're after.

Your task is to undertake at least one and preferably more self-care activities on a daily basis. It should be an activity you do for no other reason than to give yourself a chance to rest, relax, and enjoy. The activity you choose should require a not-insignificant commitment of time, so two minutes reading the newspaper doesn't count. Things that really count might include a candlelit bubble bath; curling up with a good novel; taking a walk through a quiet park or woods, meditating; playing or listening to music; or anything else that you find uniquely pleasurable. It can be an activity you do with others, if you like, but the important thing to remember is that you're trying to please yourself, not anyone else. Now, if a friend or partner can join you in your self-care activity and have a good time as well, that's great; just don't fall into your old trap of concerning yourself with others' satisfaction at the expense of your own.

It would be ideal, of course, if exercise could become a regular and pleasurable self-care activity. Norean has had success with this, because she uses her exercise time as a chance to focus only on herself. If she was so inclined she could take work with her to do while on the treadmill, since she always feels that she's running behind. But she refuses to do so, and instead spends her treadmill time doing pleasure reading. And she also makes it a point to think of no one else's needs but her own as she works out. As a result, her exercise sessions are now something she looks forward to instead of dreading them as a burdensome chore.

Self-care is a broad coping category that encompasses all the other FATS skills. Expressing feelings, setting limits, and making time for important activities could *all* be considered part of taking care of yourself, but you also need to add in the nurturing activities like those above. Giving yourself pleasure, and considering yourself a worthy recipient, are key factors in helping to rewrite old tapes and fattitudes that tell you you're not good enough.

Trena was working on her chronic bingeing. Divorced, Trena had no assistance from her ex-husband in raising their children, and she had to work full-time to make enough to support her household. As we talked about the connection between food and feelings, Trena became aware that her binges were driven in part by her loneliness and were an attempt to fill the empty space she didn't feel safe enough to fill up with a new romantic relationship. When she tried to replace her bedtime binges with self-care activities, she found herself resisting the change. As we talked about her difficulty doing something exclusively for her own pleasure, she began to cry as she related her feeling that she didn't deserve good things. This feeling was connected to her guilt over leaving her husband, despite the fact he'd been physically abusive to her on a too-regular basis. Once Trena was able to recognize she'd made a courageous decision instead of a selfish one, she was able to gradually substitute self-care activities for her binges.

Becoming adept at taking care of yourself is the

best thing you can do in the long run for your health and emotional well-being. Keep up the hard work.

SUPPORTERS AND SABOTEURS

You've already identified key support people whose assistance would be beneficial to your success. You've also identified those who get in your way. Now is the time to reorganize your social network and maximize your chances of making the progress you want to make.

Look over the Support Solicitation Form (or forms) you completed earlier. Your task now is to create an opportunity to practice your assertiveness skills by sitting down with a target support person(s) and sharing the form with them. Help them learn about what you're doing and why, and what they can do to help you. Help them learn about what not to do as well. Use this as an opportunity to ask for what you need and explain what you don't need. Show them this book if necessary and help them understand your fattitudes. Make sure you give specific examples of how your support person(s) could be helpful.

Rachel had a unique situation. She'd been married for about eight years, with no children, and her weight gain had been steady since her wedding day. Her husband, who also struggled with weight, was very supportive of her no matter what she weighed. Whenever she attempted to lose weight, he'd go along with the program. She ate low fat; he ate low fat. She exercised; he exercised. She fell off track; he fell off track. In her counseling sessions we explored what obstacles she ran into whenever she began to lose weight. What she discovered was that her husband's supportiveness was actually part of her problem: She felt "crowded" whenever she tried to reach her weight-loss goals, as if she were carrying both her *and* her husband's success on her shoulders. It was too much of a burden for Rachel. When she sat down with her husband to discuss what he could do to help her, she ended up telling him that she needed him to do *less* than he'd always done. She needed space to do her weight management work without feeling as if she were the "leader of the pack." Her husband understood, and realized that although they could be mutually supportive in their respective efforts to slim down, *he* had to take responsibility for his own progress.

You will probably face more of a challenge with your saboteurs. Recall that the success of your plan of action relies largely on whether you can change the saboteurs in your network. For those you can change, it's time to have a conference similar to the one that you have with your supporters. You might try using the same Support Solicitation Form as a way to organize your thoughts. In this instance, you'll probably be giving critical feedback about your saboteur's past and present behavior. As we discussed previously, this is one of the more difficult assertiveness challenges. Make sure you practice in advance if you feel anxious about what you have to say, which is to be expected.

Communicating with saboteurs may help them learn to change their behavior and its resulting negative impact on you. You may have to communicate your needs and feelings repeatedly, because saboteurs rarely change based on a single request. Saboteurs have a vested interest in your failure because it serves their psychological needs. Asking them to change means they face as formidable a task as you do. You're asking them to face their own fattitudes, something they may or may not be ready to do. After you've talked with your saboteurs, take time to reflect on what happened. Did you say what you wanted to say? What did you leave out? How was your message received? What else needs to be addressed? Also, remember to pat yourself on the back for taking a communication risk. Natalie took such a risk.

Natalie faced a formidable challenge in her efforts to pare down her 245 pounds. She'd been overweight for much of her childhood and had tried repeatedly to diet without any lasting success. Her parents had always been overinvolved with her weight and her eating habits. Her father had always been very critical of her appearance, and had gone so far as to force her to "weigh-in" every Saturday during her teens to assess her progress with dieting. Natalie entered therapy while she was still in college and living with her parents. Her father continued to say nasty and hurtful things when she started a new exercise program, such as "You've never lost weight before, what makes you think you can lose it now?"

Natalie categorized her father as a saboteur she could change, probably because she fantasized that he could someday become the type of father she'd always wished she'd had. She planned to have a talk with him, but felt she couldn't do it on her own, so she invited her parents to a family session. At the meeting, Natalie was very courageous in expressing her feelings toward her father's critical comments and rejecting attitude. Her father seemed to listen, but later it became clear that little had sunk in. Although he backed off as requested for a period of a few weeks, he gradually returned to his previous sabotaging behavior. Natalie tried again to ask for the support she needed, but her father was recalcitrant. It took another family session to drive home the point that her father needed to look at his own problems instead of focusing on Natalie's. The lesson here is that, again, it may require repeated communications before your saboteurs finally "get the message."

For saboteurs that you can avoid, by all means take a path around them as much as possible. It's an easy solution when available to you. If you lose nothing by reducing your contact with a saboteur, or can manage the loss, then treat yourself to the isolation. Kara did herself just such a favor by making a minor adjustment in her work schedule.

Kara discovered via her Food-Feelings Logs that she had an overwhelming urge to binge after arriving home from work. The trigger wasn't her clerical job, although she found it to be stressful at times; what really bothered her was the ride home with a coworker who lived in her neighborhood. After reflection, Kara became aware that she found the coworker (who was overweight and ate candy bars in the car) to be a very dominating, opinionated woman who allowed no disagreement and who used the ride-home time to ventilate her personal frustrations about the workday.

Kara came to realize that her binges upon arriving home were related to her squelched anger and resentment at being used as a "chew toy" by her driving companion. With this insight, Kara was able to negotiate a schedule change with her boss so that she came in later and stayed later, eliminating the sabotaging impact of commuting with her unpleasant acquaintance. Affording herself the quiet drive to and from work was a big step toward revamping her entire lifestyle.

Probably the most difficult of all are the saboteurs that you can't control and can't lessen your involvement with. What do you do? Well, the best thing is to insulate yourself to the best extent possible. Try to find support elsewhere to counteract or at least buffer the saboteur's impact. Rethink the situation to minimize the importance of the saboteur's behavior. These are all very difficult options that are clearly easier written than they are done, but it's important to remember that even if a saboteur is not within your control, you still have options. One example of this very complicated situation comes from

Vicky, a married mother of two who came to counseling for help with her longstanding history of yo-yo dieting. As we worked together it became clear that Vicky's husband had some involvement with her failure. On the outside, her husband was a saintly hardworking man, but at home tended to blame Vicky for everything that went wrong in the family and marriage. Her husband needed to maintain a focus on Vicky's problems and weaknesses because it obscured his own. She invited him to join her for marital sessions, but he refused. Vicky did not want to consider separation or divorce because of concerns for the children and her own financial viability, so she considered herself "stuck" with the situation. Her resolve to succeed was strong, though, and she refused to give up her efforts to lose weight. She was able to go outside the marriage for social support from friends, but what was really helpful was her ability to focus on the needs of her children to have a healthy role model as a way to keep herself going. Her husband tried everything he knew to knock her off track, but failed.

THE FATTITUDES FOCUS SESSION:
PHASE THREE

Your daily focus session should continue to be a part of your schedule. What you'll probably find is that you start off like gangbusters and make progress, then your effort falls off as you begin to neglect the behaviors that are getting you somewhere, and eventually you lose sight of where you're going. The focus session is a way to keep from derailing your weight-loss efforts and stay on track. Remember to do your standard tasks (see page 125 for a refresher).

In addition, pay particular attention to your efforts to master the FATS skills. Ask yourself, what problem situations did I address today? What did I do differently that led to success? You might try using the following format to guide your thinking and writing.

You should be well on your way to changing your old habits. But remember that everybody makes progress at a different rate. Don't give up if you begin to feel impatient with yourself. Keep up the hard work. Your consistent efforts will pay off in the end.

To review, during the Extinguish phase you should be doing the following self-help things:

- Use cheat sheets to help you identify and foil your fattitudes

- Take action to apply FATS to problem situations in your life

- Write unsent letters to help resolve troublesome issues from your past and present

- Take action to cultivate support and decrease the negative impact of saboteurs

JOURNAL ENTRY FORM

Today I expressed my feelings by

Today I asserted myself by

Today I managed my time better by

I took care of my own needs today by

SEVEN

"T" Is for Transform

Here we are, approaching the final stage of the Fattitudes DIET and change process. You've done a lot of work so far. Hopefully you've begun the healing process and are ready for the next step. The final step, for many, is the hardest one to take and maintain.

Let's talk about what you've done up to this point. You've taken the plunge and have looked yourself and your feelings right in the face. You've identified your emotional obstacles to healthy living. You've confronted the unresolved issues that lead to the payoffs of your pounds. You've taken the risk to try new things and to reinvent your coping style. By now you may feel like you've gotten somewhere with your inner issues.

But what about the outside? What about weight loss? What do you do now to shed the pounds you no longer need?

PHASE FOUR: *TRANSFORM*

One of my clients summed up her long process of emotional change and healing by saying, "I'm to the point now that weight management is *emotionally uncomplicated*." What she meant is that after confronting her demons and facing them down, she was now free to make the choice to eat right and exercise, something she'd never been able to do in the past because her fattitudes got in the way. And, hopefully, you're now at the same or a similar spot, because the final step in the DIET process is to **Transform** new insights and healing into healthy living.

Emotional healing is a major part of the overeating cure, but it's not entirely sufficient. True, if you disconnect food and feelings and find alternate ways of coping, you may lose weight simply because your caloric intake declines. I've seen that happen many, many times. If it happens for you, that's wonderful! To maximize your weight management success and improve your overall health, however, you must establish new eating and exercise habits. Take the emotional changes you've made and turn them into lifestyle changes.

The good news is that you already know everything you need to know about what to do next. Your years of dieting have helped you learn about healthy nutrition, and your repeated failures at keeping a regular exercise routine have taught you how to move your body to burn fat. Now, you just need to do it.

YOUR FATTITUDE-FREE MISSION STATEMENT

To guide your new lifestyle you need a set of goals called a "mission statement." A mission statement reflects your overall purpose, and should include specific means for you to accomplish your goals. Try creating one for yourself. You can use the following format if you like.

It's important to keep your mission statement close at hand as a way of organizing and motivating your efforts. After you've done the emotional work, you've still got to tackle the strength of habits and reprogram your behaviors so you can adopt new ways of doing things. Before I began a regular program of exercise I enjoyed getting up in the morning and waking up by reading the newspaper and drinking a cup of coffee. The impetus to live a healthier lifestyle and to establish an exercise habit came primarily from the consultation work I was doing with cardiac rehabilitation patients. I saw the serious and life-threatening effects of bad habits and decided I'd better learn to eat right and exercise so I wouldn't have someone sawing open my chest at some point in the future. I committed myself to lowering my fat intake (which meant Burger King for lunch three days a week just *had* to go) and getting frequent aerobic activity.

I was busy, just like everyone else: I worked full time and was married, and back then we were dealing with our first child and all that that meant. When I got home from work there were many things that demanded my time and attention. I realized that if I wanted to be successful at regular exercise, I needed to get it done in the morning. Consequently, I decided I had to modify my morning routine. I had to give up my leisurely perusing of the headlines over a steaming cup of java in favor of sweating on the treadmill. It wasn't easy, but I had to do it. And you can, too.

Fattitudes

FATTITUDE-FREE MISSION STATEMENT

My overall goal in changing my lifestyle is

To accomplish this goal I need to

To maintain my progress, each day I have to

I intend to reward my progress and maintain my commitment by

I'll know I'm doing well when I

BUT WHAT DO I EAT?

If you took time to read everything there is in print today about nutrition and weight loss, you'd probably end up skinny because you'd be exhausted, frustrated, and confused. There's an overabundance of expert advice on what to eat and what not to eat these days, but there's little, if any, agreement among our authorities. One says eat a lot of protein and minimal carbohydrates. Another says eat little protein and a lot of carbohydrates. Our government tells us to eat inside a pyramid. But, then again, our government was telling us something quite a bit different about twenty-five years ago. Maybe twenty-five years from now, they'll tell us another truth. And then there are the dozens of full-page newspaper ads that tell us to eat whatever we want, but just take this fat-absorbing pill or that herbal supplement, and the pounds will burn away all by themselves. So even the well-informed might still feel in the dark about how to choose the right foods.

Does Fattitudes have the key to what to eat and when? No, we're not going to offer you a food plan or a set of surefire recipes. We don't hold ourselves out as nutritional experts. Besides, research has shown that individuals tend to do better with losing weight and keeping it off if they create their *own* nutritional plan. If you do it yourself, you'll feel more like it's your own, and ownership is a crucial ingredient to commitment.

Almost every dietitian we've consulted with over the years has pointed out the importance of *balance*. Too much or too little of anything is unhealthy. That's also true in psychology: Most of the "answers" to life lie somewhere in the happy medium or near the "golden average." The best thing about eating a "balanced" diet is that no foods are forbidden if eaten in moderation and if the overall equation doesn't equal "too much" of either calories or fat. The most important thing to remember when planning your food choices is to continue to be aware of any remaining connections between food and feelings, and to avoid a "diet mentality" at all cost. Don't let yourself fall into old dieting traps that lead to deprivation and frustration. By all means, don't fall prey to quick-fix expectations and the destructive impatience that they create.

Some people do well by trying to change one eating habit at a time, like dropping a "nemesis food" (i.e., one that is your downfall) or beginning by planning one meal a day to be your "healthy" one. Others need to tackle the whole issue at one time. The key is to decide what's best for *you*. Think about your own needs and situation. What's reasonable? What changes have the best chance of success? Make your plan. Break it down into step-by-step segments, then begin. Remember to reward yourself for attaining short-term goals, and keep your mind off the goal weight or the ultimate outcome.

If you feel a need for some outside assistance, as many still do even after doing a lot of emotional work, then by all means consult a local expert. Call a lifestyle change studio to help you with your nutritional plan. Consult your physician for referrals or guidance. Find a registered dietitian who has a good reputation in your community. But, stay away from gimmicky programs that make unrealistic claims and who merely see you as a cash cow for their bottom line.

WHAT'S THE RIGHT WAY TO EXERCISE?

Things are a bit more clear-cut when creating an optimal exercise program, because in the area of exercise science, there's a lot more agreement about what we should do. The research is overwhelmingly clear about the health benefits of regular exercise: In our modern society it's the closest thing we have to a "cure-all." It's also the most potent factor in promoting long-term weight management success. Overall, exercise is the best thing you can do for yourself to enhance both your physical and your emotional well-being.

There's a long laundry list of what exercise does for your health: It helps prevent cardiac disease and cancer, boosts our resistance to illness, and reduces stress. It's a weapon against anxiety and depression, and helps prevent diabetes. Exercise also helps keep us from losing our memories and other cognitive abilities as we get older, slows down the aging process, and promotes clearer thinking and creativity.

What exercise does for weight loss is also substantial. If you combine regular aerobic activity with strength training, you'll speed up your metabolism and burn fat even more quickly. You'll gradually replace fat with muscle tissue, which takes up less space and uses up more calories on a daily basis, even when you're at rest. You'll tone up, firm up, and maintain your bone density as you get older, so fractures and osteoporosis will be less likely.

Most experts say that daily activity is best. Thirty to forty-five minutes per day is a good target, as long as you engage in exercise that is of sufficient intensity to get your heart rate into a "training range." What's your training range? Take your age and subtract it from 220. Then multiply the result by sixty percent to get the bottom of your range, and by eighty-five percent to get the top of your range. Your heart rate per minute should be somewhere toward the middle of your training range to get the best cardiovascular benefit.

Even a little exercise is better than none at all. And furthermore, it's never too late to start. Studies have shown significant improvement in endurance, lung capacity, and cardiovascular fitness for those who begin a regular low-impact exercise program, even if they've never exercised in the past.

Although aerobic activities are fairly straightforward and easy to understand, strength training is an undertaking that often requires some education, because the risk of injury is much higher. If you have access to—and can afford—a qualified personal trainer, that's great. Go for it! Even if you can't, most community recreation facilities or Ys have staff available to assist you in properly using weights. A personal trainer can also be a great aid in maintaining your motivation and commitment.

At the very least, get an exercise buddy; it can be very helpful. Just don't let your association with a buddy fertilize your fitness fattitudes (e.g., "My buddy's out of town so I'll take a week off, too").

When you're using strength training and exercise as a primary component of your weight management efforts, don't let the scale fool you. Don't let "pounds lost" be the only measure of progress or the absence thereof. When you're building muscle mass your inches will go down but your weight might stay the same or even increase. Make sure you avoid "weight equals worth" fattitudes. We've gotten so wedded to the scale as a measure of success that almost everyone has a bathroom scale. It's so easy to climb on top of it every day to get some indication of how we're doing, but it's such a trap! The lesson to learn is to keep your eyes on health as a goal. Healthy weight management will be a by-product of your efforts if you do.

MOTIVATIONAL TIPS AND TRICKS

Since lifestyle change requires such a concerted effort, one of the keys to accomplishing it is motivation. Where do you get your motivation? How do you maintain your motivation when the going gets rough? There are many ways to accomplish this task, and many people come up with creative solutions to keep themselves on track. There was a recent research study that showed people who kept a picture of their clogged arteries (taken during a cardiac examination) in their billfolds or purses had greater success over the long term with reducing cholesterol and weight. Not many of us have access to such a picture, but perhaps there are other more feasible techniques you can use. To get you started, we've gathered a list of tips for motivation maintenance:

Keep a picture of your "before" weight in a prominent place

Reward yourself for each small health accomplishment

Schedule workouts on a weekly planner

Call an exercise buddy when feeling a motivational lag

Write down positive self-statements and keep them with you

Buy a gorgeous outfit in a smaller size and keep it in your closet

Make a chart of your exercise progress using colors and bar graphs

Watch a favorite TV show or video while exercising

Celebrate your "wins"

Hire a personal trainer

Exercise with a group of like-minded individuals

Think about your kids and setting a good example

Imagine aging as a vigorous and youthful you

Send yourself postcards with encouraging words

Get someone else to send you postcards with encouraging words

Look at each bead of sweat as another dose of immunity from illness

Find success stories in magazines, books, or on the Internet

Join a weight management discussion and support group—in person or in cyberspace

This is only a small list of things that we know have worked for many people. What's really important is finding what works for you. When you find it, use it!

STILL FEELING STUCK?

You may have read this far and done everything asked of you, but still feel like you're getting nowhere fast. I've run into this situation many times with clients, who seem to be working very hard at changing but remain in the same unhappy spot. Whenever this occurs, ninety-nine percent of the time the obstacle is an undiscovered payoff for being overweight, or a steadfast fear of changing. If you're not moving forward, there's a reason for it, and your task is to find it before you brand yourself hopeless. One helpful technique is, once again, to take out pen and paper and write an essay entitled "Why I'm Choosing to Remain Fat and Miserable." The results might surprise you, especially if you take responsibility for your "stuckness" and figure out what else needs to be done.

It's important to point out, though, that even if you're doing the right things and are making progress with finding, fighting, and foiling your fat-titudes, you may feel like you're going in the wrong direction. It is a common occurrence among those who are working on beating emotional eating to gain weight before being able to turn things around. Why? Because digging into hurts often feels like sticking your hand into a hornet's nest. Plus, changing is stressful, and in times of stress we often fall back to our old ways of coping. The old adage in psychotherapy is that you may well begin to feel worse before you begin to feel better. The same is true for self-help efforts.

One of the most frequently encountered obstacles to progress is feeling trapped by hurts and traumas from the past. A common question is, "How do I get over my childhood? It happened so long ago!" Healing childhood hurts is a major problem for some, especially if the hurts have been severe and prolonged. There's no easy solution, unfortunately. What's key is forgiveness. Forgiveness of those you hold responsible for what happened to you, but also forgiveness of yourself. Stop holding on to the emotional notion that you only got what you deserved. It's so common for children to personalize the blame for their own neglect and abuse, because they're unable to see the situation objectively. They're unable to say to themselves something like "Daddy's got a problem with his self-esteem and he drinks too much because he's in so much pain. That's why he hits me.

It's not because I'm no good." If we could say those things, we might be able to insulate ourselves from the hurt that tends to follow us as we grow up. It's only by feeling compassion for ourselves that we're able to begin to heal and love ourselves.

Laurie had been coming to counseling for about eight months. She had worked very hard at digging up her fattitudes and trying to improve self-esteem, but she remained in a rut of depression and overeating. Much of her efforts both in and out of session had been to work on grieving over the loss of a happy childhood. One day she came to session, with a brighter expression on her face, and announced, "I've gone ahead and gotten a personal trainer." I was shocked and pleased, because she'd always avoided any steps toward change, and this was a big one. When I asked her what had prompted her to make such a decision, she said very simply, "I just got sick of myself being this way. I'm sitting around in this depressive funk, crying over losing my past, when all I'm doing is depriving myself of a future." She'd finally gotten over her fear of changing, and decided she may as well take some risks and live. She knew she'd probably run into snags and issues along the way, but planned to work them out in her counseling sessions.

If you're still sitting on or near square one, you

may not be ready to risk changing because of everything it brings up. If so, give yourself some more time, and whatever you do, don't succumb to the "What's the use, why bother?" fattitudes that are so destructive. You deserve more.

If your self-help efforts falter, don't be reluctant to get some consultation and consider professional assistance. A savvy psychotherapist can be a valuable aid in attacking lifelong patterns of self-defeating behavior. Anne says it best:

> *I always had a nagging feeling while sitting in the consultation room of a weight-loss center that something was missing in the plan. They knew what I should eat, they knew what I should not eat, but none of them really asked me why I was eating. But in the Fattitudes group I found the missing piece to the puzzle: a group of women of different weights, stories, and issues, but with a common bond in our emotional dependence on food. As a result, I no longer feel alone in my struggle. With the help of my group members I have learned more about myself and the meaning behind my eating than I thought was possible. Instead of coming "out of the closet" as they say, I have come "out of the refrigerator."*

RELAPSE PREVENTION

Even if you've done a lot of work and feel like you're on track to healthy living, you should expect to hit some bumps along the way. The path to success is often winding and pitted with chuckholes, so you should have a relapse prevention plan in mind ahead of time. For example, you may very well be in a groove with exercising and eating right, for a stretch of several weeks, then "something happens" and you've lost your motivation and commitment, and the whole program goes to pot. When that happens, it's important to figure out what that "something" was that knocked you down. Retrace your steps. Think back over the time preceding your derailment. What was going through your mind? What were you feeling? Did a fattitude sneak in? Did somebody say or do something that was sabotaging?

Janice had been doing very well with her exercise plan for about a month, then one session came in and was bewildered by her complete regression to her old ways. She'd stopped exercising and had even binged a few times in the week since our last session. By retracing her steps, she discovered that a comment made by a coworker that "too much exercise is bad for you" had sapped Janice's commitment to healthy living and led to her backslide.

Sometimes it doesn't take much to throw us off. These "fattitude fits," when old issues get triggered and we fall back into old patterns of thinking and feeling, can be very demoralizing. What do you do in this situation? Well, the solution to a fattitude fit is to *focus*. That means, focus on what happened to cause the fit, then focus on your goals and your success strategies so you can get back on track. Nobody makes lifestyle change without encountering frustrations along the way, so don't kick yourself if you get into the same pickle.

Robin was honest with herself when she identified that she'd often fall off course in her weight management efforts because of the tremendous pressure she felt to return to using food for emotional coping. One day she said,

Food continues to be a tempting refuge for me. It's the only thing in my life I've always felt completely in control of. When I can't get what I need from other people, food just seems like something that's available to me in limitless supply. Food is abundant! It's everywhere! I can find whatever I need whenever I need it. Food never stands me up for a date. Cheeseburgers never send me mixed messages, or lie to me, or tell my secrets to some-

one else. I can feel like I'm an "interpersonal anorexic" but still find company in a chocolate bar. The level of trust I have in food is just really hard to replace.

The message here is, changing a long-standing pattern of eating to meet emotional needs is something that requires consistent effort. Don't beat yourself up for hitting what seems like a dead end along the way.

THE FATTITUDES RECIPE FOR SUCCESS

To tie things together, here's a concise summary of what we consider to be the ten most essential elements of a successful weight management plan. Let this "recipe" be an overall guide for your change efforts:

- **TAKE PERSONAL RESPONSIBILITY FOR YOUR HEALTH.** The only person you can rely on to do what's necessary is yourself. It sounds obvious, but many times we tend to blame external factors for throwing us off track. Don't let it happen.

- **FOCUS ON PERMANENT, NOT TEMPORARY CHANGES.** What you're after is a permanent new you, rather than trying to change a long-term problem with short-term efforts. Remember the rule of thumb: Don't do anything on a diet you're not willing to do the rest of your life.

- **CLEAR YOUR MOTIVATION OF FATTI-TUDES.** Recognize that the universal obstacle to healthy weight management is self-defeating behavior. Work on being your own best friend instead of your own worst enemy.

- **SET REALISTIC, STEP-BY-STEP GOALS.** As comedian Bill Murray said in the movie *What About Bob?* the key to change is "baby-stepping." Focus on short-term hurdles instead of gazing longingly at the finish line.

- **STRENGTHEN FATS TO FIGHT FAT.** The crucial importance of Feelings expression, Assertiveness, Time management, and Self-care cannot be overemphasized. Work on these skills to make life more manageable and to decrease your reliance on food for emotional coping.

- **CULTIVATE AND UTILIZE YOUR SUPPORT NETWORK.** Lifestyle change almost always requires help from supportive others. Ask for what you want, and return the favor when someone else needs it from you. Try to insulate yourself against those saboteurs who want you to fail because it meets *their* needs.

- **FOCUS ON EXCERSIZE AS THE KEY TO LONG-TERM MAINTENANCE.** Research has shown again and again how important regular physical activity is to weight management and health in general. Work on making exercise an "addiction" you're proud to have.

- **DEVELOP AND MAINTAIN NONFOOD METHODS OF SATISFYING YOUR NEEDS.** Ending a lifelong reliance on food for fun and coping can be a formidable challenge. Look around you at other options and push yourself to find other feel-good activities. Recognize the *choice* involved in overeating.

- **GET YOUR INSPIRATION WHEREVER YOU CAN.** Nothing inspires success like someone else's success. Read magazines. Find Internet chats. Let your role models show you the way.

- **EXPECT RELAPSES IN TIMES OF STRESS.** Lifestyle change is never complete. Don't sweat the missteps and stumbles, and don't beat yourself for wrong turns. Focus on where you want to go and remember the map you've created for yourself.

THE FATTITUDES FOCUS SESSION:
PHASE FOUR

Your focus session should continue to be a regular part of your daily schedule. Even after you get some success under your belt, keep up with your journals. Take a look back over the weeks and months of your DIETing and note the little bits and pieces of insight you've collected along the way. How has your thinking changed? How have your feelings changed? What obstacles remain in your way? What was most helpful? What do you need to do more of to continue to progress?

If you've fallen off track with your journals, look at it as evidence of self-sabotage. Ask yourself why you've stopped doing something that is very potent for producing change. Don't let your commitment to yourself slip away!

EIGHT

•

A FINAL WORD

JEFF: As we've said over and over again, finding, fighting, and foiling your fattitudes is one of the toughest jobs anyone will ever face. It's frustrating, and at times it feels utterly hopeless. It often seems so much easier just to surrender and get used to being miserable. What's key is not to give up, because everyone is different. People make progress at different rates, and can get stuck in the mud along the way.

NOREAN: I certainly did. Progress is usually uneven, too. For a long time I thought I was stuck in the "T" stage, knowing what I should do, and thinking that I just wasn't able to make the commitment to exercising and eating right. What I didn't know, though, was that I still had some "discovering" to do. Once I found those last few fattitudes, the path to health was a lot easier to find. Then, what I needed was to focus on my long-term motivators to keep me going.

I remember two incidents in particular that really brought this home in a big way. I was driving along with Evan, then two and a half, in the backseat and he spied a man jogging along the road. He said, "Look, Mommy, that man is working out like you do." I was so thrilled by this, because I'm not a runner, but he still recognized his mommy's efforts. Then, the plum came from our daughter Allison. One day after I'd been exercising regularly for a couple of months Allie came to me and asked, "Mommy, do you lose weight when you work out?" I replied, "Yes," not knowing where the conversation was going. Then she said, "I just wondered because now I can get my arms around you when I hug you." That really got to me. I think about that little comment whenever I run into a motivational lag. It's what keeps me going.

JEFF: Your progress hasn't been easy.

NOREAN: Far from it. I've had to work really intensely at staying on top of things. One of the biggest obstacles I ran into, especially early on in my efforts to change my eating and exercise habits, was impatience. I still wished everything would hurry up. I expected to be just like one of those fitness magazine and infomercial success stories, you know, six months to a new body.

JEFF: You weren't losing weight fast enough.

NOREAN: No, I wasn't. There I was, working out and sweating and doing everything right, but where was the magical payoff? I didn't see any major changes in the mirror the first few months, and the scale didn't drop like I expected, so I had a lot of trouble keeping up with my routine. I was making fairly steady progress with losing inches and dropping fat, which showed up in my dress size decreasing, but I was still too centered on weight loss. Everything was happening way too slowly.

JEFF: I remember when Norean hit one of those frustrating weight-loss plateaus early on, and it seemed like her progress had come to a grinding halt. She sent me the following E-mail from work one day:

Having been raised to look at the scale and constantly getting asked how much I lost, I find it very difficult to still be looking at 219! For God's sake when I started this crap I was at 250, maybe. I was 230ish when I started Just Results. That's less than 11 pounds in 10 months. One pound a month and I'm doing 20 times more now than I did before I started! It's real hard not to give up. I keep pushing harder and harder and I can't get anywhere near dropping under 200 and into size 16. I really don't think I'm asking for much here. Sometimes I just want to hurt something or someone because I'm so frustrated!!! If my trainer wasn't bigger than me and bench-pressed my weight, I'd have to hurt him.

OK, that was quite a bit of venting. However, I truly am losing it sometimes. I'm running out of ways to feel good about this when nothing is changing. I wish I could find another type of motivation since obviously size change isn't hap-pening, weight loss ain't ever gonna happen, and I can't see or feel the health changes.

NOREAN: Yes, I remember that one all too well. I've had to deal with frustration like that all along the way. With my genetic structure, it seems like I've had to scrape and scrounge for every inch and pound of progress. My body requires almost twice as much cardiovascular activity as the "average" person does to speed up metabolism enough to make a dent in my weight. Jeff's support has been invaluable because I've been so demoralized at times that I've wanted to pitch the whole she-bang.

JEFF: I can be supportive now in ways I couldn't be supportive in the past. I know that sounds odd, since I'm supposed to be a professional helper, but when my own personal demons were stirred up, it was hard to be objective. I've had to confront this very issue with my clients who learned of this book and our personal struggles with weight, which I had never disclosed before. The reactions were quite varied. Some were pleased to learn that I really knew what the pain was all about since I'd dealt with it at close range. Others felt ashamed that they were still struggling with issues my wife had conquered. And still others felt confused when they learned about my history of being critical of my wife for being overweight. They wondered how I could be sensitive to *their* insecurities and self-hatred given how I'd felt in the past. I basically admitted that, yes, I sounded like a professional hypocrite. How could I be in the role of helper to others when I'd been unable to be helpful to my wife all those years? One client was really upset fearing that I'd been secretly repulsed by her weight when I'd appeared to be so accepting. The truth is that I have *never* felt critical of one of my clients. But it's different when you're personally involved. I'm human, and being human I've made some mistakes in my personal life. It's because of my personal struggles that I've tried to learn so much about this problem as a professional. I would have handled things between Norean and me a lot differently if I'd known years ago what I know now.

NOREAN: Like you said, when you're involved in an intimate relationship, the demons come alive like nowhere else.

JEFF: That's right. So, let's try to sum up. Looking back, I'm curious about what you'd say you've learned from all this.

NOREAN: Well, the biggest thing was to learn not to expect the quick fix. It's something I still struggle with. The magic cure doesn't exist. I looked for it for years and just got more and more discouraged about my weight. I didn't want to acknowledge that weight management requires a lot of hard work and a lifetime commitment. I also realize now that I'll always have to listen to my inner voice to prevent future sabotage. I'll have to stay focused and remind myself of my long-term goals and keep using the support system I have. I have to remind myself that progress comes as slowly and as surely as the weight gain did. I guess the best way to put it is that given the demons that have plagued my weight management efforts, the bottom line for me is a combination of *exercising* and *exorcising*.

That's the biggest lesson for me. What about you? What have you learned?

JEFF: Tons. The most pointed lesson is how one partner's personal demons can wreak havoc on the other. People can really destroy each other if they don't realize what they're doing. And another lesson is that I can't solve your problems for you. I can be supportive of your efforts, but it's not something I have any control over. Every time I tried to control it in the past, all I did was make things worse.

NOREAN: I had to find the answer on my own. Not that outside help wasn't helpful, but I had to find my own style. I broke the problem down and tackled things one at a time. That worked for me. It might not work for anyone else.

JEFF: Any last-minute advice for our readers?

NOREAN: Giving advice is so tricky. Over the years I've received—and ignored—advice from hundreds of expert sources. I heard what I was ready to hear when I was ready to hear it. So many people presumed they knew what to tell me. But they didn't. Like, I love the "justs." Any advice that begins with "just" is basically worthless. "Just push yourself away from the table." Or "just exercise." If it were really that easy, it wouldn't be a problem for so many of us.

JEFF: I used to say a lot of "justs," didn't I?

NOREAN: Yes. You did.

JEFF: You know, it sounds like it's a wonder we made it.

NOREAN: We were close to divorce more than a few times.

JEFF: I remember dividing up the property on paper at least once.

NOREAN: Back when all we had to worry about was who got the cat.

JEFF: I *never* worried about who got the cat.

NOREAN: Yeah, we've been through a lot.

JEFF: But at the risk of sounding a little hokey, I think we're closer now than we've ever been.

NOREAN: I agree.

JEFF: We stuck it out, and our love and connection to each other has kept us going.

NOREAN: I guess the most important thing is that we worked at it—and found our way through.

ONE LAST TASK

As a final exercise, we want you to write *your* story. Write down the details of your struggle, hopefully with the aid of those who've been involved. Let it tell about who you are and where you've been, and most important, where you're going. What fattitudes did you uncover? How did you foil them? What obstacles did you encounter? What keeps you going? When you're finished, make a copy and send one to us at P.O. Box 79, Springboro, Ohio, 45066, or via E-mail to Stories@fattitudes.com. We'd love to hear from you!